Biosynthetic Products for Cancer Chemotherapy

Volume 3

Biosynthetic Products for Cancer Chemotherapy

Volume 3

George R. Pettit

and

Richard H. Ode
Arizona State University, Tempe

PLENUM PRESS · NEW YORK AND LONDON

Library of Congress Cataloging in Publication Data

Pettit, George R
    Biosynthetic products for cancer chemotherapy.

    Vol. 2 by G. R. Pettit and G. M. Cragg; Vol. 3 by G. R. Pettit and R. H. Ode.
    Includes bibliographies and indexes.
    1. Cancer – Chemotherapy. 2. Antineoplastic agents. I. Cragg, Gordon M. L.
[DNLM: 1. Neoplasms – Drug therapy. 2. Antineoplastic agents; QZ267 P511b]
RC271.C5P47   616.9′94′061   78-54146
ISBN 0-306-40095-2 (v. 3)

© 1979 Plenum Press, New York
A Division of Plenum Publishing Corporation
227 West 17th Street, New York, N.Y. 10011

Printed in the United States of America

Preface

Fortunately the scientific and medical literature related to cancer chemotherapy is now expanding rapidly. While this is most excellent for future cancer treatment prospects, it is becoming more difficult for all the researchers in chemotherapy—bio-organic chemists involved with the discovery of new anticancer drugs, biologists and pharmacologists developing these new drugs, and physicians doing the clinical research—to keep abreast of current achievements in these disciplines so vitally important to effective cancer treatment. The purpose of Volumes 1 and 2 of this work was to provide useful reviews of current progress in discovery and clinical application of new biosynthetic cancer chemotherapeutic drugs. Volume 1 gave a general view of the cancer problem and cancer treatment using biosynthetic products, based on literature available through December 1975. Volume 2 included mainly the first summary of plant and animal biosynthetic antineoplastic and/or cytotoxic constituents to April 1976.

The survey comprising this third volume has been divided into two sections. Section A provides an extension of the Volume 2 data on plant and animal antineoplastic and/or cytotoxic constituents to July 1977. The introduction to Section A brings the summary of such biosynthetic products to literature available November 1, 1977. Section B incorporates a summary of data of essentially all previously isolated and characterized marine animal constituents irrespective of biological activity. The rapidly increasing likelihood that clinically useful cancer chemotherapeutic drugs will be isolated from marine animals suggested that a relatively complete synopsis of marine animal biosynthetic products known through July 1977 would be especially timely and useful to a broad cross section of chemists and biologists. The outline of Section B was begun some seven years ago when our Cancer Research Institute programs began to routinely require such information. It is hoped that the result will now be helpful to all chemists and biologists concerned with marine animal chemistry. When the preparation of Section B was initiated, no such summary was available and this situation obtained until 1976 when the very useful but less detailed work of Baker and Murphy became available.[26] Their work covers marine animal and marine plant constituents through 1973.

v

In Section B our attempts at locating all pure and characterized marine animal components for the past approximately 100 years has probably not been perfect. Some compounds were no doubt missed and we extend our apologies to anyone affected by such oversights and other possible errors in this volume. We appreciate very much the assistance of Drs. T. R. Kasturi, P. R. Reucroft, and T. B. Harvey, III with some early literature studies needed for preparation of the marine animal data. Grateful appreciation is also extended to Mrs. Christine H. Duplissa for general and expert assistance with preparation of the data and to Mrs. Marie Baughman and Miss Melinda A. Duplissa for very helpful aid in final manuscript preparation.

George R. Pettit
Paradise Valley, Arizona
November, 1977

Contents

Section A. *New Biosynthetic Antineoplastic and/or Cytotoxic Agents: Tabular Survey* 1

Introduction 3

Chapter 1. Higher Plant Terpenoids 9

Chapter 2. Higher Plant Steroids 17

Chapter 3. Higher Plant Lignans 19

Chapter 4. Quinones, Flavans, and Other Nonnitrogenous Higher Plant Products 21

Chapter 5. Higher Plant Alkaloids, Amides, and Ansa Macrolides . 27

Chapter 6. Fungi and Other Lower Plant Biosynthetic Products . 35

Chapter 7. Marine Invertebrate and Other Lower Animal Biosynthetic Products 41

Chapter 8. Marine Vertebrate and Other Higher Animal Biosynthetic Products 43

Section B. *Marine Animal Biosynthetic Products* 45

Introduction 47

Chapter 9. Hydrocarbons, Alcohols, and Esters 61

Chapter 10. Sterols and Steroids 65

Chapter 11. Terpenoids 87

Chapter 12. Carbohydrates 125

Chapter 13. Phenols, Quinones, and Related Compounds . . . 127

Chapter 14. Amino Acids. 145

Chapter 15. Amines and Nitrogen Heterocyclic Compounds . . 151

Subject Index

Section A

(*A*) *Higher Plants* 175

(*B*) *Higher Plant Components* 175

(*C*) *Fungi and Other Lower Plants* 176

(*D*) *Fungi and Other Lower Plant Components* 176

(*E*) *Marine Invertebrates and Other Lower Animals* 176

(*F*) *Marine Invertebrate and Other Lower Animal Biosynthetic Products* 176

(*G*) *Marine Vertebrates and Other Higher Animals* 176

(*H*) *Marine Vertebrate and Other Higher Animal Biosynthetic Products* 176

Section B

(*A*) *Marine Animals* 176

(*B*) *Marine Animal Components* 178

Molecular Weights

   (*A*) *Plants* 182

   (*B*) *Marine Animals* 182

Bibliography 185

Section A
New Biosynthetic Antineoplastic and/or Cytotoxic Agents: Tabular Survey

Introduction

The U.S. National Cancer Institute's program, begun in 1957, directed at isolation of naturally occurring antineoplastic agents, has amply demonstrated that certain plants and animals do indeed produce a great variety of anticancer agents. In recent years the dramatic discoveries arising from this program have stimulated a great deal of interest and initiation of analogous programs on a worldwide basis. This fortunate series of events is now allowing new antineoplastic and/or cytotoxic biosynthetic products to be discovered at an increasing rate. Very illustrative are the 487 antineoplastic and/or cytotoxic compounds described in Volume 2 of this series, which covers the literature to April 1976. In this section of the present volume are listed 99 compounds appearing in the literature from that date to July 1977. The following three-month period to November 1977 yielded more new results that will be briefly summarized here and eventually incorporated in a subsequent volume.

Before we begin a summary of the most recent advances, two important reviews of plant antineoplastic and cytotoxic constituents need to be cited. Cordell and Farnsworth[105] have summarized their recent studies concerning the isolation of plant anticancer agents and have prepared a broader review of plant anticancer agents appearing in the 1974–1976 period.[104] A specific treatment of structure/activity relationships in the colchicine area has been prepared by Kiselev.[233] Most importantly, a complete issue of the 1976 *Cancer Treatment Reports* was devoted to recent status of the National Cancer Institute's higher and lower plant programs. The summaries and conclusions of Hartwell (higher plant constituents),[175] Spjut and Perdue (primitive medical plant leads),[397] Douros (lower plant constituents),[113] Wall *et al.* (isolation techniques),[425] Smith *et al.* (homoharringtonine),[393] Kupchan (mechanisms of action),[255] and Carter and Livingston (clinical trials)[72] are particularly noteworthy.

The following outline of advances appearing in the literature over the three-month period August–November 1977 provides an illustration of current efforts to discover new higher and lower plant cancer chemotherapeutic drugs. In 1973, we reported the first pseudoguaianolide-type sesquiterpene to display *in vivo* antineoplastic activity.[328,330] At that time, we found the sesquiterpene lactone helenalin to be quite active against the

3

P388 lymphocytic leukemia (T/C 220 at 3 mg/kg) and the Walker 256 carcinoma (subcutaneous, 47 to 58% inhibition at 1.5 to 3 mg/kg). Subsequently helenalin was found to be the active antineoplastic constituent of several compositae, the most recent being *Anaphalis morrisonicola* Hay.[273] Helenalin has been shown to inhibit DNA synthesis and DNA polymerase enzyme action in Ehrlich ascites tumor cells.[272] Similarly, two other known active sesquiterpene lactones, costunolide and parthenolide, have been isolated from *Michelia champaca* and *Talauma ovata*.[182] The cytotoxic agents of *Bursera klugii* (Burseraceae) were found to be sapelin A and sapelin B.[209] The major cytotoxic and antineoplastic constituent of

Sapelin A
PS: T/C 136 (5 mg/kg)
Reference 209

Sapelin B
PS: T/C 138 (1.25 mg/kg)
Reference 209

Simarouba versicolor (Simaroubaceae) was shown to be the known quassinoid-type terpene glaucarubinone.[159] A very simple cytotoxic constituent, namely 2,6-dimethoxybenzoquinone, was isolated from the pantropical *Xylosma velutina* (Flacourtiaceae).[103] The Farnsworth group has also

2,6-dimethoxybenzoquinone
KB: ED$_{50}$, 2.8 μg/ml
Reference 103

isolated the dieneone jacaranone from twig-leaf and stem bark from the Columbian plant *Jacaranda caucana* Pittier (Bignoniaceae).[316] Three new

Jacaranone
PS: T/C 165 (2 mg/kg)
PS: ED$_{50}$, 1.3 μg/ml
References 105, 316

possibly cytotoxic diterpenoids bearing 2-pyrone ring systems have been isolated from *Podocarpus nagi*.[177] In the lignan area 5′-desmethoxydeoxy-podophyllotoxin has been characterized as the active component of

5′-Desmethyldeoxypodophyllotoxin
PS: T/C 127 (50 mg/kg)
KB: ED_{50}, 4 × 10^{-4} μg/ml
Reference 208

Bursera morelensis (Buseraceae).[208] In addition the known deoxypodo-phyllotoxin was isolated again from *Juniperus bermudiana* (Pinaceae).[406]

Among the nitrogen-containing plant biosynthetic products, the indole alkaloids continue to receive major emphasis. The previously known tubotaiwine *N*-oxide was found to be the cytotoxic component of *Tabernae-montana holstii* K. Schum. (Apocynaceae).[231] The same plant has been

Tubotaiwine *N*-Oxide
PS: ED_{50}, 1.8 μg/ml
KB: inactive
Reference 231

found to yield the bisindole alkaloid gabunine as a companion cytotoxic constituent.[232] Kutney and colleagues[264] have continued to develop excellent synthetic approaches to the clinically important bisindole alkaloids vincristine and vinblastine. For example, catharanthine *N*-oxide and vindoline have been condensed in the presence of trifluoroacetic anhydride at low temperatures to yield 3′,4′-dehydrovinblastine.[268] Kutney *et al.*[266,270] have devised a very useful synthesis of the antineoplastic bisindole alkaloid leurosine based on analogous Polonovoski-type coupling between 3β,4β-epoxy-3,4-dihydrocatharanthine N_b-oxide with vindoline. Synthesis of 3′-hydroxyvinblastine[266] has been completed and methods have also been devised recently for obtaining other modifications of the vinca alkaloids.[265,267,269] A review of the ergot-type indole alkaloids as possible prolactin and mammary cancer inhibitors has been prepared by Cassady

Gabunine
PS: ED$_{50}$, 3.2 μg/ml
Reference 232

and Floss.[73] The most significant recent advance involving the nitrogen-containing macromolecules has been purification of the glycoprotein cesalin from the seeds of *Caesalpinia gilliesii* Wall.[304]

A potentially useful model for drug design based on structure/activity relationships among the higher plant antineoplastic agents has been summarized by Moore.[306] The concept of bioactivation as one mechanism for drug action was extended to the assumption that certain naturally occurring antineoplastic drugs may undergo reduction *in vivo* to yield a potent alkylating unit. Such bioreductive alkylating agents would contain olefin systems capable of undergoing Michael-type addition reactions by nucleophiles.

The lower plants have continued to be a fruitful source of antineoplastic biosynthetic products. From the anthracycline mixture produced by an *Actinosporangium* sp. Nettleton *et al.* have isolated and characterized two new antitumor antibiotics, namely, musettamycin and marcellomycin.[313] Attempts have also been made to carry out microbiological transformations of daunomycinone[213] and Arcamone[23] has synthesized an interesting variety of daunomycin and adriamycin derivatives and related anthracyclines. The previously known antibiotic vermiculine from *Pencillium vermiculatum* Dangeard[186] has been shown to be cytotoxic to HeLa and L5178Y cells. A related study of some well-known commercial antibiotics using murine L1210 cells showed tetracycline to be the most cytotoxic followed by erythromycin, clindamycin, chloramphenicol, and cephaloglycin.[279] The new anticancer antibiotics of unknown structure include PSX-L (very active against L1210 murine lymphocytic leukemia).[154] PO-357 from a *Streptosporangium* sp. (a basic polypeptide of molecular weight 8500–9000)[419] and SS-228 Y from an Actinomycetales of marine origin.[239,320] Doubtlessly, the marine muds will prove to be an excellent

Musettamycin

Marcellomycin

Antineoplastic activity
Reference 313

source of potentially useful antineoplastic agents.[320,324] A very helpful review concerned with the production and structural elucidation of the bleomycins and phleomycins has been prepared by Umezawa.[418]

The new antineoplastic and/or cytotoxic agents appearing in the literature over the period April 1976 through July 1977 have been collected in Chapters 1–8. The data have been arranged as in Volume 2 of this series.[329] The plant and animal antineoplastic and/or cytotoxic agents have been grouped according to natural products chemistry classification and biosynthetic origin and arranged in order of increasing carbon atom content within each group. The data include, where known, a structure, a common name, the system and results of antineoplastic screening and/or cytotoxicity evaluations, a melting point and optical rotation value, whether certain spectral data have been reported, and finally the organism of origin and reference. A compilation of the better known *in vitro* and *in vivo* anticancer screening systems and criteria for significant activity (for the most commonly employed) used by the National Cancer Institute have been entered in the appendix of Volume 2.[329]

Chapter 1

Higher Plant Terpenoids

$C_{14}H_{16}O_3$ **Mexicanin-E**

MOL. WT.: 232
MELTING POINT: 95–100°C
$[\alpha]_D$: −55   SOLVENT: Chf
SPECTRAL DATA: IR, PMR
ORGANISM: *Helenium microcephalum* (Compositae)
LOCATION: Texas
REFERENCE: 275

$C_{15}H_{18}O_4$ **Microhelenin-A**

MOL. WT.: 262
BIOACTIVITY: Walker 256
          T/C, 148 (2.5 mg/kg)
MELTING POINT: 140–141°C
$[\alpha]_D$: +89   SOLVENT: Me
SPECTRAL DATA: PMR, Mass Spec
ORGANISM: *Helenium microcephalum* (Compositae)
REFERENCE: 274

$C_{18}H_{18}O_6$ **Samaderin A**

MOL. WT.: 330
BIOACTIVITY: KB and PS: Inactive
MELTING POINT: 253–255°C
$[\alpha]_D$: −31.3   SOLVENT: Py
SPECTRAL DATA: UV, IR, PMR, Mass Spec
ORGANISM: *Samadera indica* (Simaroubaceae)
REFERENCE: 426

$C_{20}H_{24}O_6$ Enmein

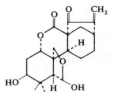

MOL. WT.: 360
BIOACTIVITY: Ehrlich ascites
               Increase in life span, 66%
ORGANISM: *Isodon japonicus* and *Isodon trichocarpus*
               (Labiatae)
REFERENCE: 151

$C_{20}H_{26}O_3$ Jatrophatrione

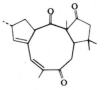

MOL. WT.: 314
MELTING POINT: 148–150°C
$[\alpha]_D$: −187   SOLVENT: Chf
SPECTRAL DATA: UV, IR, PMR, Mass Spec
ORGANISM: *Jatropha macrorhiza* Benth. (Euphorbiaceae)
REFERENCE: 409

$C_{20}H_{26}O_4$ Stemolide

MOL. WT.: 330
MELTING POINT: 235–237°C
SPECTRAL DATA: UV, IR, PMR, Mass Spec
ORGANISM: *Stemodia maritima* (Scrophulariaceae)
REFERENCE: 285

$C_{20}H_{26}O_5$ Microhelenin-C

MOL. WT.: 346
MELTING POINT: Gum
$[\alpha]_D$: −85.0   SOLVENT: Me
SPECTRAL DATA: IR, PMR, Mass Spec
ORGANISM: *Helenium microcephalum* (Compositae)
LOCATION: Texas
REFERENCE: 275

$C_{20}H_{26}O_8$ Samaderin E

MOL. WT.: 394
BIOACTIVITY: KB and P388: Moderate activity
MELTING POINT: 202–207°C; Diacetate, 267–270°C
$[\alpha]_D$: −11.7   SOLVENT: Py
SPECTRAL DATA: UV, IR, PMR, Mass Spec
ORGANISM: *Samadera indica* (Simaroubaceae)
REFERENCE: 426

$C_{20}H_{28}O_5$ Microhelenin-B

MOL. WT.: 348
MELTING POINT: 111–113°C
$[\alpha]_D$: −84.9   SOLVENT: Me
SPECTRAL DATA: IR, PMR, Mass Spec
ORGANISM: *Helenium microcephalum* (Compositae)
LOCATION: Texas
REFERENCE: 275

$C_{20}H_{28}O_6$ Oridonin

MOL. WT.: 364
BIOACTIVITY: Ehrlich ascites
                    Increase in life span, 115%
ORGANISM: *Isodon japonicus* and *Isodon trichocarpus*
                    (Labiatae)
REFERENCE: 151

$C_{21}H_{30}O_{10}$ Penstemide

MOL. WT.: 442
BIOACTIVITY: PS: T/C, 184 (50 mg/kg)
SPECTRAL DATA: UV, IR, PMR
ORGANISM: *Penstemon deutus* Dougl. ex Lindl.
                    (Scrophulariaceae)
REFERENCE: 207

$C_{24}H_{34}O_7$ **Trichokaurin**

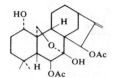

MOL. WT.: 436
BIOACTIVITY: Ehrlich ascites
   Increase in life span, 17%
ORGANISM: *Isodon japonicus* and *Isodon trichocarpus*
   (Labiatae)
REFERENCE: 151

$C_{25}H_{30}O_7$ **Phyllanthocin**

MOL. WT.: 442
BIOACTIVITY: KB: ED_{50}, 10^{-2} μg/ml
MELTING POINT: 126–127°C
$[\alpha]_D$: +25.2   SOLVENT: Chf
SPECTRAL DATA: UV, PMR, Mass Spec
ORGANISM: *Phyllanthus brasiliensis* (Muell.) (Euphorbiaceae)
LOCATION: Costa Rica
REFERENCE: 259

$C_{25}H_{34}O_9$ **Simalikalactone D**

MOL. WT.: 478
BIOACTIVITY: PS: T/C, 165–175 (4–1 mg/kg)
   KB: ED_{50}, 10^{-2}–10^{-3} μg/ml
ORGANISM: *Quassia amara* L. (Simaroubaceae)
REFERENCE: 262

$C_{27}H_{36}O_{11}$ **Quassimarin**

MOL. WT.: 536
BIOACTIVITY: PS: T/C, 165–175 (4–1 mg/kg)
   KB: ED_{50}, 10^{-2}–10^{-3} μg/ml
MELTING POINT: 237.5–238.5°C
$[\alpha]_D$: +22.4   SOLVENT: Chf
SPECTRAL DATA: UV, IR, PMR, Mass Spec
ORGANISM: *Quassia amara* L. (Simaroubaceae)
REFERENCE: 262

$C_{28}H_{50}O_{11}$ Baccharin

MOL. WT.: 562
BIOACTIVITY: PS: T/C, 200 (1.25–5.0 mg/kg)
KB: ED_{50}, 10^{-3}–10^{-4} μg/ml
MELTING POINT: 200–230°C
$[\alpha]_D$: +41.5   SOLVENT: Chf
SPECTRAL DATA: UV, IR, PMR, Mass Spec
ORGANISM: *Baccharis megapotamica* Spreng
(Asteraceae)
REFERENCE: 256

$C_{30}H_{48}O_3$ Betulinic Acid

MOL. WT.: 456
BIOACTIVITY: PS: T/C, 135 (100 mg/kg)
T/C, 140 (50 mg/kg)
MELTING POINT: 284–286°C
SPECTRAL DATA: IR, PMR, Mass Spec
ORGANISM: *Vauquelinia corymbosa* Correa (Rosaceae)
REFERENCE: 410

$C_{30}H_{48}O_3$ Ursolic Acid

MOL. WT.: 456
BIOACTIVITY: PS: T/C 125 (50 mg/kg)
MELTING POINT: 288–291°C
$[\alpha]_D$: +60
SPECTRAL DATA: IR, PMR, Mass Spec
ORGANISM: *Vauquelinia corymbosa* Correa (Rosaceae)
REFERENCE: 410

$C_{30}H_{50}O_2$ Uvaol

MOL. WT.: 442
BIOACTIVITY: PS: T/C, 125 (100 and 200 mg/kg)
MELTING POINT: 224–225°C
SPECTRAL DATA: IR, PMR, Mass Spec
ORGANISM: *Vauquelinia corymbosa* Correa
(Rosaceae)
REFERENCE: 410

$C_{32}H_{46}O_{10}$　　**Gnidiglaucin**

MOL. WT.: 590
$[\alpha]_D$: +36　　　　　SOLVENT: Chf
SPECTRAL DATA: UV, IR, Mass Spec
ORGANISM: *Gnidia glaucus* Fres. (Thymelaeaceae)
REFERENCE: 261

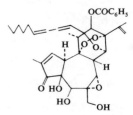

$C_{37}H_{44}O_{10}$　**Gnidilatidin**

MOL. WT.: 648
$[\alpha]_D$: +28　　　　　SOLVENT: Chf
SPECTRAL DATA: UV, IR, Mass Spec
ORGANISM: *Gnidia latifolia* Gilg. (Thymelaeaceae)
REFERENCE: 261

$C_{37}H_{48}O_{10}$　**Gnidilatin**

MOL. WT.: 652
BIOACTIVITY: PS: T/C, 130–140
　　　　　　　P388: ED$_{50}$, 20–80 μg/kg
$[\alpha]_D$: +52　　　　　SOLVENT: Chf
SPECTRAL DATA: UV, IR, Mass Spec
ORGANISM: *Gnidia latifolia* Gilg. (Thymelaeaceae)
REFERENCE: 261

$C_{40}H_{52}O_{17}$　**Phyllanthoside**

(2 × 6-Deoxyglucose)

MOL. WT.: 804
BIOACTIVITY: PS: T/C, 137–153 (6–24 mg/kg)
　　　　　　　KB: Inactive
MELTING POINT: 125–126°C; Pentaacetate, 114–117°C
$[\alpha]_D$: +19.2　　　　　SOLVENT: Chf
SPECTRAL DATA: UV, IR, PMR
ORGANISM: *Phyllanthus brasiliensis* (Muell.) (Euphorbiaceae)
LOCATION: Costa Rica
REFERENCE: 259

$C_{44}H_{54}O_{12}$ Gnidimacrin

MOL. WT.: 774
BIOACTIVITY: PS: T/C, 180
             P388: ED_{50}, 12–16 μg/kg
MELTING POINT: 172–174°C
$[\alpha]_D$: −3.9   SOLVENT: Chf
SPECTRAL DATA: UV, IR, PMR, Mass Spec
ORGANISM: *Gnidia subcordata* Meissn. Engl. (Thymelaeaceae)
REFERENCE: 260

$C_{53}H_{74}O_{11}$ Gnidilatidin 20-palmitate

MOL. WT.: 886
BIOACTIVITY: PS: T/C, 170
             P388: ED_{50}, 2–0.5 μg/kg
$[\alpha]_D$: +27   SOLVENT: Chf
SPECTRAL DATA: UV, IR, Mass Spec
ORGANISM: *Gnidia latifolia* Gilg. (Thymelaeaceae)
REFERENCE: 261

$C_{53}H_{78}O_{11}$ Gnidilatin 20-palmitate

MOL. WT.: 890
BIOACTIVITY: PS: T/C, 170
             P388: ED_{50}, 2–0.5 μg/kg
$[\alpha]_D$: +45   SOLVENT: Chf
SPECTRAL DATA: UV, IR, Mass Spec
ORGANISM: *Gnidia latifolia* Gilg. (Thymelaeaceae)
REFERENCE: 261

$C_{60}H_{84}O_{13}$ Gnidimacrin 20-palmitate

MOL. WT.: 1012
BIOACTIVITY: PS:T/C, 190
             P388: ED_{50}, 30–50 μg/kg
$[\alpha]_D$: −1.5   SOLVENT: Chf
SPECTRAL DATA: UV, IR, PMR, Mass Spec
ORGANISM: *Gnidia subcordata* Meissn. Engl.
             (Thymelaeaceae)
REFERENCE: 260

Higher Plant Steroids

$C_{34}H_{48}O_{14}$ **Hyrcanoside**

MOL. WT.: 680
BIOACTIVITY: PS: T/C, 133 (1.25 mg/kg)
            KB: ED_{50}, 0.1, 0.7 μg/ml
MELTING POINT: 205–208°C
SPECTRAL DATA: UV, IR, PMR
ORGANISM: *Coronilla varia* L. (var. penngift)
            (Leguminosae)
REFERENCE: 442

Higher Plant Lignans

$C_{21}H_{20}O_7$ 4′-Demethyldeoxypodophyllotoxin

MOL. WT.:   384
BIOACTIVITY: PS: T/C, 132 (2.1 mg/kg)
       KB: ED_{50}, $1.2 \times 10^{-3} \mu g/ml$
MELTING POINT: 246–248°C
SPECTRAL DATA: IR, PMR, Mass Spec
ORGANISM: *Polygala macradenia* Gray (Polygalaceae)
LOCATION: Texas
REFERENCE: 183

$C_{23}H_{22}O_5$ Isouvaretin

MOL. WT.:   378
BIOACTIVITY: KB: ED_{50}, 1.9 $\mu g/ml$
       P388, ED_{50}, 1.9 $\mu g/kg$
MELTING POINT: Gum
SPECTRAL DATA: UV, IR, PMR, Mass Spec
ORGANISM: *Uvaria chamae* (Annonaceae)
LOCATION: Ghana
REFERENCE: 271

$C_{23}H_{22}O_5$ Uvaretin

MOL. WT.:   378
BIOACTIVITY: PS: T/C, 133 (10 mg/kg)
MELTING POINT: 162–163°C
SPECTRAL DATA: UV, IR, PMR, Mass Spec
ORGANISM: *Uvaria cucuminata* Oliv. (Annonaceae)
REFERENCE: 100

$C_{23}H_{22}O_5$ Uvaretin

BIOACTIVITY: mono-Me: T/C, 132 (1 mg/kg)
               di-Me: T/C, 144 (4 mg/kg)
               T/C, 141 (2 mg/kg)
MELTING POINT: 138–139°C; 122–123°C
ORGANISM: *Uvaria cucuminata* oliv. (Annonaceae)
REFERENCE: 100
BIOACTIVITY: KB: ED_{50}, 1.0 μg/ml
               P388: ED_{50}, 1.0 μg/kg
MELTING POINT: 164–165°C
SPECTRAL DATA: UV, IR, PMR, Mass Spec
ORGANISM: *Uvaria chamae* (Annonaceae)
LOCATION: Ghana
REFERENCE: 271

$C_{30}H_{28}O_6$ Diuvaretin

MOL. WT.:   484
BIOACTIVITY: KB: ED_{50}, 2.0 μg/ml
               P388: ED_{50}, 0.84 μg/kg
MELTING POINT: Gum
SPECTRAL DATA: UV, IR, PMR, Mass Spec
ORGANISM: *Uvaria chamae* (Annonaceae)
LOCATION: Ghana
REFERENCE: 271

Chapter 4

Quinones, Flavans, and Other Nonnitrogenous Higher Plant Products

$C_9H_6O_3$ Umbelliferone

MOL. WT.: 162
BIOACTIVITY: KB: ED_{50}, 33 $\mu g/ml$
MELTING POINT: 223–224°C
SPECTRAL DATA: UV, IR PMR, Mass Spec
ORGANISM: *Coronilla varia* L. (var. penngift) (Leguminosae)
REFERENCE: 442

$C_9H_{10}O_4$ Jacaranone

MOL. WT.: 182
BIOACTIVITY: PS: T/C, 165 (2 mg/kg)
            KB: ED_{50}, 2.1 $\mu g/ml$
MELTING POINT: 53–54°C
SPECTRAL DATA: UV, IR, PMR, Mass Spec
ORGANISM: *Jacaranda caucana* Pittier (Bignoniaceae)
LOCATION: Colombia
REFERENCE: 317

$C_{15}H_{10}O_5$ Aloe emodin

MOL. WT.: 270
BIOACTIVITY: PS: T/C, 133–154 (20 mg/kg)
MELTING POINT: ·223–224°C
ORGANISM: *Rhamnus frangula* L. (Rhamnaceae)
REFERENCE: 257

$C_{15}H_{12}O_4$ Pinocembrin

MOL. WT.:   256
BIOACTIVITY: KB: ED_{50}, 21 μg/ml
                        P388: ED_{50}, 10.5 μg/kg
MELTING POINT: 194–195°C
SPECTRAL DATA: UV, IR, PMR, Mass Spec
ORGANISM: *Uvaria chamae* (Annonaceae)
LOCATION: Ghana
REFERENCE: 271

$C_{16}H_{14}O_4$ Pinostrobin

MOL. WT.:   270
MELTING POINT: 109–110°C
SPECTRAL DATA: UV, IR, PMR
ORGANISM: *Uvaria chamae* (Annonaceae)
LOCATION: Ghana
REFERENCE: 271

$C_{17}H_{14}O_6$ 3,5-Dihydroxy-4′,7-dimethoxyflavone

MOL. WT.:   314
BIOACTIVITY: KB: ED_{50}, 3.0 μg/ml
MELTING POINT: 229–231°C
SPECTRAL DATA: UV, IR, PMR, Mass Spec
ORGANISM: *Lychnophora affinis* Gardn. (Compositae)
LOCATION: Brazil
REFERENCE: 278

$C_{17}H_{14}O_7$ 3,6-Dimethoxy-4′,5,7-trihydroxyflavone

MOL. WT.:   330
BIOACTIVITY: PS: Inactive
                        KB: Inactive
                        P388: ED_{50}, 3.4 μg/kg
MELTING POINT: 198–200°C
SPECTRAL DATA: UV, IR, PMR, Mass Spec
ORGANISM: *Acanthospermum glabratum* (D.C) Wild (Compositae)
LOCATION: Tanzania
REFERENCE: 353

$C_{18}H_{16}O_6$ **5-Hydroxy-3′,4′,7-trimethoxyflavone**

MOL. WT.:   328
BIOACTIVITY: KB: ED_{50}, > 1.00 $\mu g/ml$
MELTING POINT: 166–168°C
SPECTRAL DATA: UV, IR, PMR, Mass Spec
ORGANISM: *Lychnophora affinis* Gardn. (Compositae)
LOCATION: Brazil
REFERENCE: 278

$C_{18}H_{16}O_7$ **4′,5-Dihydroxy-3′,7,8-trimethoxy-flavone**

MOL. WT.:   344
BIOACTIVITY: KB: ED_{50}, > 10 $\mu g/ml$ (low solubility)
MELTING POINT: 163–166°C
SPECTRAL DATA: UR, IR, PMR, Mass Spec
ORGANISM: *Lychnophora affinis* Gardn. (Compositae)
LOCATION: Brazil
REFERENCE: 278

$C_{18}H_{18}O_2$ **Juncusol**

MOL. WT.:   266
BIOACTIVITY: KB: ED_{50}, 0.3 $\mu g/ml$
MELTING POINT: 176°C; Diacetate, 110°C
SPECTRAL DATA: IR, PMR, Mass Spec
ORGANISM: *Juncus roemerianus* (Juncaceae)
LOCATION: Mississippi
REFERENCE: 292

$C_{19}H_{12}O_7$ **Daphnoretin**

MOL. WT.:   352
BIOACTIVITY: KB: ED_{50}, 43 $\mu g/ml$
MELTING POINT: 246–247°C
SPECTRAL DATA: UV, IR, PMR, Mass Spec
ORGANISM: *Coronilla varia* L. (var. penngift) (Leguminosae)
REFERENCE: 442

$C_{19}H_{18}O_7$ 5-Hydroxy-3',4',7,8-tetra-
               methoxyflavone

MOL. WT.: 358
BIOACTIVITY: KB: ED_{50}, $> 100 \; \mu g/ml$
MELTING POINT: 155–158°C; Acetate, 176–180°C
SPECTRAL DATA: UV, IR, PMR, Mass Spec
ORGANISM: *Lychnophora affinis* Gardn. (Compositae)
LOCATION: Brazil
REFERENCE: 278

$C_{19}H_{18}O_8$ 3',5-Dihydroxy-4',5',7,8-
               tetramethoxyflavone

MOL. WT.: 374
BIOACTIVITY: KB: ED_{50}, $> 10 \; \mu g/ml$
MELTING POINT: 141–146°C
SPECTRAL DATA: UV, IR, PMR, Mass Spec
ORGANISM: *Lychnophora affinis* Gardn. (Compositae)
LOCATION: Brazil
REFERENCE: 278

$C_{19}H_{24}O_6$ Tagitinin F

MOL. WT.: 348
BIOACTIVITY: PS: T/C, 161–155 (50–12.5 mg/kg)
MELTING POINT: 128–130°C
$[\alpha]_D$: -144
SPECTRAL DATA: UV, IR, Mass Spec
ORGANISM: *Tithonia tagitiflora* Desf. (Compositae)
REFERENCE: 321

$C_{22}H_{18}O_5$ Chamanetin

MOL. WT.: 362
BIOACTIVITY: KB: ED_{50}, $5.2 \; \mu g/ml$
               P388: ED_{50}, $2.4 \; \mu g/kg$
MELTING POINT: 210–211°C
SPECTRAL DATA: UV, IR, PMR, Mass Spec
ORGANISM: *Uvaria chamae* (Annonaceae)
LOCATION: Ghana
REFERENCE: 271

$C_{22}H_{18}O_5$ Isochamanetin

MOL. WT.: 362
BIOACTIVITY: KB: ED_{50}, 2.4 $\mu g/ml$
             P388: ED_{50}, 2.2 $\mu g/kg$
MELTING POINT: 215–217°C
SPECTRAL DATA: UV, IR, PMR, Mass Spec
ORGANISM: *Uvaria chamae* (Annonaceae)
LOCATION: Ghana
REFERENCE: 271

$C_{29}H_{24}O_6$ Dichamanetin

MOL. WT.: 468
BIOACTIVITY: KB: ED_{50}, 1.2 $\mu g/ml$
             P388: ED_{50}, 1.4 $\mu g/kg$
MELTING POINT: 118–120°C
SPECTRAL DATA: UV, IR, PMR, Mass Spec
ORGANISM: *Uvaria chamae* (Annonaceae)
LOCATION: Ghana
REFERENCE: 271

Polysaccharide F-1

BIOACTIVITY: Ehrlich ascites carcinoma
             20 mg/kg
             10 of 10 survived 60 days
ORGANISM: *Sargassum thunbergii* (Phaeophyta)
             (Fucales Order)
REFERENCE: 202

Polysaccharide F-2

Polysaccharide

BIOACTIVITY: Active against Sarcoma 180
ORGANISM: *Coriolus versicolor* (Basidiomycetes—Class)
REFERENCE: 181

Chapter 5

Higher Plant Alkaloids, Amides, and Ansa Macrolides

$C_{20}H_{16}N_2O_4$ **Camptothecin**

MOL. WT.: 348
ORGANISM: *Ophiorrhiza mungos* Linn.
(Rubiaceae)
LOCATION: S.E. Asia
REFERENCE: 405

$C_{21}H_{18}N_2O_5$ **10-Methoxycamptothecin**

MOL. WT.: 378
BIOACTIVITY: 10 times better against herpes virus than camptothecin
Antiviral
Herpes virus
100% and 89% inhibition of plaques
20 and 10 ng/ml
ORGANISM: *Ophiorrhiza mungos* Linn. (Rubiaceae)
LOCATION: S.E. Asia
REFERENCE: 405

$C_{35}H_{34}N_2O_5$ Trilobine

MOL. WT.:   562
BIOACTIVITY: HeLa-S_3: ED_{50}, 1.1 μg/ml
REFERENCE: 263

$C_{36}H_{36}N_2O_5$

MOL. WT.:   576
BIOACTIVITY: HeLa-S_3: ED_{50}, 2 μg/ml
                           EAC: 30
                           S-180: 25
                           LD_{50}, 115
REFERENCE: 263

$C_{36}H_{36}N_2O_6$ Cepharanoline

MOL. WT.:   592
BIOACTIVITY: HeLa: ED_{50}, > 30 μg/ml
REFERENCE: 263

$C_{36}H_{38}N_2O_6$ Hypoepistephanine

MOL. WT.:   594
BIOACTIVITY: EAC: Inactive
                           HeLa: ED_{50}, 12 μg/ml
REFERENCE: 263

$C_{36}H_{38}N_2O_6$ Stebisimine

MOL. WT.: 594
BIOACTIVITY: HeLa: ED_{50}, 16 $\mu g/ml$
REFERENCE: 263

$C_{37}H_{38}N_2O_6$ Cepharanthine

MOL. WT.: 606
BIOACTIVITY: EAC: 30
            S-180: 100
            LD_{50}: 125
            HeLa: ED_{50}, 5.5 $\mu g/ml$
REFERENCE: 263

$C_{37}H_{40}N_2O_6$ Berbamine

MOL. WT.: 608
BIOACTIVITY: EAC, S-180: Inactive
            HeLa-S_3: ED_{50} > 10 $\mu g/ml$
            LD_{50}: 75
REFERENCE: 263

$C_{37}H_{40}N_2O_6$ Epistephanine

MOL. WT.: 608
BIOACTIVITY: EAC: Inactive
            HeLa: ED_{50}, 14 $\mu g/ml$
REFERENCE: 263

$C_{37}H_{40}N_2O_6$ Fangchinoline

MOL. WT.: 608
BIOACTIVITY: EAC: Inactive
            LD_{50}: > 50
            HeLa: ED_{50}, 4.1 $\mu g/ml$
REFERENCE: 263

$C_{37}H_{40}N_2O_6$ Thalicberine

MOL. WT.: 608
BIOACTIVITY: S-180: Inactive
EAC: 62.5
LD_{50}: > 125
HeLa: ED_{50}, 13 μg/ml
REFERENCE: 263

$C_{37}H_{42}N_2O_6$ Cycleanine

MOL. WT.: 610
BIOACTIVITY: HeLa: ED_{50}, 12 μg/ml
REFERENCE: 263

$C_{37}H_{44}Cl_2N_2O_6$ Isoliensinine dihydochloride

MOL. WT.: 683
BIOACTIVITY: HeLa: ED_{50}, 16 μg/ml
EAC: Inactive
REFERENCE: 263

$C_{38}H_{42}N_2O_6$ 0-Methylthalicberine

MOL. WT.: 622
BIOACTIVITY: EAC: Inactive
          LD$_{50}$: 125
REFERENCE: 263

$C_{38}H_{44}N_2O_6$ Dauricine

MOL. WT.: 624
BIOACTIVITY: HeLa-S$_3$: ED$_{50}$, 10 μg/ml
          EAC: > 100
          S-180: Inactive
          LD$_{50}$: > 125
REFERENCE: 263

$C_{39}H_{46}N_2O_6$ 0-Methyldauricine

MOL. WT.: 638
BIOACTIVITY: HeLa: ED$_{50}$, 11 μg/ml
          EAC: > 100
          S-180: Inactive
          LD$_{50}$: > 125
REFERENCE: 263

C$_{39}$H$_{46}$I$_2$N$_2$O$_6$ **Oxyacanthine dimethiodide**

MOL. WT.:   892
BIOACTIVITY: HeLa: ED$_{50}$, > 30 μg/ml
                      EAC: Inactive
REFERENCE: 263

C$_{40}$H$_{46}$I$_2$N$_2$O$_6$ **Tetraandrine dimethiodide**

MOL. WT.:   904
BIOACTIVITY: EAC: Inactive
                      LD$_{50}$: 7
                      HeLa: ED$_{50}$, > 30 μg/ml
REFERENCE: 263

C$_{40}$H$_{46}$I$_2$N$_2$O$_6$ **Insularine dimethiodide**

MOL. WT.:   904
BIOACTIVITY: EAC: Inactive
                      LD$_{50}$: 10
                      HeLa: ED$_{50}$ > 30 μg/ml
REFERENCE: 263

$C_{40}H_{48}N_2O_6$ **Tetramethylmagnolamine**

MOL. WT.:   652
BIOACTIVITY: HeLa: ED_{50}, 13 μg/ml
REFERENCE: 263

Chapter 6

Fungi and Other Lower Plant Biosynthetic Products

C₅H₇ClN₂O₄   **U-43,795 (NSC-176324)**

MOL. WT.: 194
MELTING POINT: 165°C
SPECTRAL DATA: UV, IR, PMR, Mass Spec
ORGANISM: *Streptomyces sviceus* (Streptomycetaceae)
REFERENCE: 286

C₈H₁₂N₂O₃   **Primocarcin**

MOL. WT.: 184
SPECTRAL DATA: UV, IR
REFERENCE: 201, 403

$$CH_3CONHCCOCH_2CH_2CONH_2$$
$$\overset{\|}{CH_2}$$

C₈H₁₆O₇   **Usnic acid**

MOL. WT.: 224
BIOACTIVITY: PS: T/C, 135–152 (20–200 mg/kg)
ORGANISM: *Cladonia leptoclada* des.Abb.
(Cladoniaceae)
REFERENCE: 258

$C_{15}H_{18}N_2O_4$ Tomaymycin

MOL. WT.: 301
BIOACTIVITY: Active against gram-positive
Marked inhibitory effect on L1210
in vitro
MELTING POINT: Methyl ether ~145–146°C (dec.)
$[\alpha]_D$: +423   SOLVENT: Py
SPECTRAL DATA: UV
ORGANISM: *Streptomyces achromogenes* var. *tomaymyceticus*
(Streptomycetaceae)
REFERENCE: 191

$C_{16}H_{17}N_3O_4$ Anthramycin

MOL. WT.: 315
BIOACTIVITY: Wide antibacterial *in vitro*
In vivo inactive
Antitumor Sarcoma 180
Walker 256
EA
Human epidermoid carcinoma No. 3
Human adenoma No. 1
MELTING POINT: 120°C (dec.)
$[\alpha]_D$: +930   SOLVENT: DMF
SPECTRAL DATA: UV
ORGANISM: *Streptomyces refuineus* var. *thermotolerans* (Streptomycetaceae)
REFERENCE: 191

$C_{20}H_{24}O_8$ Vermiculine

MOL. WT.: 392
BIOACTIVITY: Cytotoxic antibiotic
ORGANISM: *Penicillium vermiculatum* Dangeard
(Moniliaceae)
REFERENCE: 152

$C_{24}H_{31}N_3O_7$ Sibiromycin

MOL. WT.:   473

BIOACTIVITY: Active against *Bacillus* sp., *Staphylococcus aureus*, E. coli, six transplanted mice tumors
Effective against squamous praegastric cancer cells (OG-5), ascitic forms of tumors, Sarcoma 180

MELTING POINT: 120°C (dec.)

$[\alpha]_D$:   +525   SOLVENT: DMF

SPECTRAL DATA: UV

ORGANISM: *Streptosporangium sibiricum* (Actinomycetaceae)

REFERENCE: 191

$C_{30}H_{39}NO_5$ Kodo-cytochalasin-1 (Cytochalasin H)

MOL. WT.   493

BIOACTIVITY: LD_{50}: 12.5 $\mu g/kg$

SPECTRAL DATA: PMR

ORGANISM: *Phomopsis* sp. (Unknown)

REFERENCE: 33

$C_{32}H_{36}N_2O_5$ Chaetoglobosin C

MOL. WT.:   528

BIOACTIVITY: Toxin

MELTING POINT: 257–259°C

SPECTRAL DATA: IR, PMR, Mass Spec

ORGANISM: *Penicillium aurantio-virens* Biourge (Moniliaceae)

REFERENCE: 398

MELTING POINT: 260–263°C

$[\alpha]_D$:   −30   SOLVENT: Me

SPECTRAL DATA: ·UV, IR, PMR, Mass Spec

ORGANISM: *Chaetomium globosum* (Unknown)

REFERENCE: 372

$C_{32}H_{36}O_5N_2$ Chaetoglobosin D

MOL. WT.: 528
MELTING POINT: 216°C
$[\alpha]_D$: −269   SOLVENT: Me
SPECTRAL DATA: UV, IR, PMR, Mass Spec
ORGANISM: *Chaetomium globosum* (Unknown)
REFERENCE: 372

$C_{32}H_{38}O_5N_2$ Chaetoglobosin E

MOL. WT.: 530
MELTING POINT: 279–280°C
$[\alpha]_D$: +158   SOLVENT: Me
SPECTRAL DATA: UV, IR, PMR, Mass Spec
ORGANISM: *Chaetomium globosum* (Unknown)
REFERENCE: 372

$C_{32}H_{38}O_5N_2$ Chaetoglobosin F

MOL. WT.: 530
MELTING POINT: 177–178°C
$[\alpha]_D$: −69   SOLVENT: Chf
SPECTRAL DATA: UV, IR, PMR, Mass Spec
ORGANISM: *Chaetomium globosum* (Unknown)
REFERENCE: 372

$C_{34}H_{44}N_2SO_{18}$ U-43,120 (NSC-163500)

MOL. WT.: 800
BIOACTIVITY: PS: T/C, Toxic (150 mg/kg)
                 150 (25.0 mg/kg)
                 139 (12.5 mg/kg)
       Antibiotic gram-positive, 1–2 μg/ml
       P388 and LD: ED_{50}, 2.5 μg/ml
MELTING POINT: 119–122°C
$[\alpha]_D$: +9.3   SOLVENT: Chf
SPECTRAL DATA: UV, IR, PMR
ORGANISM: *Streptomyces paulus* Dietz sp.n. (Streptomycetaceae)
REFERENCE: 173, 440

$C_{39}H_{45}NO_{16}$ Nogalamycin

MOL.WT.:   787
SPECTRAL DATA: UV, PMR
ORGANISM: *Streptomyces nogalater* var. *nogalater* sp.n. (Streptomycetaceae)
REFERENCE: 441

Unknown polysaccharide

BIOACTIVITY: Ehrlich ascites carcinoma
                16 of 20 mice had complete regression at 60 days and 20 mg/kg
ORGANISM: Culture filtrate *Fomes fomentarius* (Polyporaceae)
REFERENCE: 203

Sporamycin

ORGANISM: *Streptosporangium pseudovulgare* (No.
                PO-357) (Actinomycetaceae)
REFERENCE: 249

Neothramycins A and B

ORGANISM: *Streptomyces* sp. No. MC916-C4 (Streptomycetaceae)
REFERENCE: 191

Chapter 7

Marine Invertebrate and Other Lower Animal Biosynthetic Products

$C_{11}H_{16}O_3$ Loliolide

MOL. WT.: 196
BIOACTIVITY: P388: ED_{50}, 3.5 $\mu g/kg$
MELTING POINT: 153–154°C
SPECTRAL DATA: IR, PMR, Mass Spec
ORGANISM: *Dolabella ecaudata* (Mollusca)
REFERENCE: 335

$C_{16}H_{30}O_2$ Palmitoleic acid

$CH_3(CH_2)_5CH{=}CH(CH_2)_7CO_2H$

MOL. WT.: 254
BIOACTIVITY: P388: ED_{50}, 0.96 $\mu g/kg$
MELTING POINT: Methyl ester
SPECTRAL DATA: Mass Spec
ORGANISM: *Vespula pensylvanica* (Arthropoda/Insecta) Hymenoptera
REFERENCE: 327

$C_{18}H_{34}O_2$ Oleic acid

$CH_3(CH_2)_7CH{=}CH(CH_2)_7CO_2H$

MOL. WT.: 282
BIOACTIVITY: P388: ED_{50}, 0.67 $\mu g/kg$
MELTING POINT: Methyl ester
SPECTRAL DATA: Mass Spec
ORGANISM: *Vespula pensylvanica* (Arthropoda/Insecta) Hymenoptera
REFERENCE: 327

Chapter 8

Marine Vertebrate and Other Higher Animal Biosynthetic Products

$C_{20}H_{34}O_5$ **Prostaglandin E_1**

MOL. WT.: 370
BIOACTIVITY: B1 cell line growth inhibition
REFERENCE: 355

60-Unit protein

```
    1
Leu-Lys-Cys-Asn-Lys-Leu-Val-Pro-
        10
Leu-Phe-Tyr-Lys-Thr-Cys-Pro-Ala-Gly-
        20
Lys-Asn-Leu-Cys-Tyr-Lys-Met-Phe-Met-
            30
Val-Ser-Asn-Leu-Thr-Val-Pro-Val-Lys-
            40
Arg-Gly-Cys-Ile-Asp-Val-Cys-Pro-Lys-
            50
Asn-Ser-Ala-Leu-Val-Lys-Tyr-Val-Cys-
            60
Cys-Asn-Thr-Asp-Arg-Cys-Asn
```

BIOACTIVITY: LD_{50}: 56 $\mu g/ml$
Yoshida sarcoma: ED_{50}, 7.4 $\mu g/ml$
ORGANISM: *Naja naja atra* (Chordata/Reptilia) Formosan cobra
REFERENCE: 212

Sphyrnastatin 1 (glycoprotein)

BIOACTIVITY: PS: T/C, 120 (1.25 mg/kg)
ORGANISM: *Sphyrna lewini* (Chordata/Pisces) Sphyrnidae
REFERENCE: 338

Sphyrnastatin 2 (glycoprotein)

BIOACTIVITY: PS: T/C, 144 (15 mg/kg)
ORGANISM: *Sphyrna lewini* (Chordata/Pisces) Sphyrnidae
REFERENCE: 338

Strongylostatin 1 (glycoprotein)

BIOACTIVITY: PS: T/C, 153 (10 mg/kg)
ORGANISM: *Strongylocentrotus drobachiensis* (Echinodermata)
REFERENCE: 332

Strongylostatin 2

BIOACTIVITY: PS: T/C, 131 (8 mg/kg)
ORGANISM: *Strongylocentrotus drobachiensis* (Echinodermata)
REFERENCE: 332

Section B
Marine Animal Biosynthetic Products

Introduction

Marine organisms represent a vast available resource for new drugs of use in medicine. However, this exceedingly valuable natural resource has been subject to surprisingly little of the bio-organic chemical investigation necessary to discover new drugs. Fortunately, this situation is rapidly changing for the better and we hope that the survey of marine animal constituents prepared for this section will enhance progress, especially in the isolation and characterization of new marine animal antineoplastic and/or cytotoxic components. A history and rationale for this approach to developing new cancer chemotherapeutic drugs has already been provided in Volume 1 of this series.[325] A recent summary of marine-organism-derived drugs for a broad range of medical problems has been made by Grant and Mackie.[165] Some of the better-known clinical advances include the isolation of cephalosporin C produced by a fungus isolated from an ocean sewage outfall. A related example is the bromine-containing anti-fungal agent thelepin related to griseofulvin.[179] The pyrrolidine derivative kainic acid obtained from the red algae *Digenia simplex* is being used in Japan as an effective anthelmintic for intestinal worms.[417] Another interesting clinical example entails the use of tetrodotoxin as an analgesic and muscle relaxant in patients with cancer and neurogenic leprosy.[318,352] Most importantly, adenine arabinoside (ara-A) was first synthesized and characterized as part of the National Cancer Institute's program directed by Baker in 1960,[276] which was based on the valuable leads provided by the earlier isolation of 1-β-D-arabinofuranosyl derivatives of thymine (spongo-thymidine)[37] and uracil (spongouridine)[38] from the Caribbean sponge *Cryptotethya crypta*. Ara-A [80,176,357,402] has proved to be the treatment of choice for the usually fatal human viral disease herpes encephalitis. The human mortality rate from herpes simplex encephalitis is about 70% and it fell to 28% in the initial clinical trial of this first truly curative agent for human viral disease.[439] Of course, cytosine arabinoside (ara-C), a well-known cancer chemotherapeutic drug, was also developed from the early lead presented by these sponge nucleoside arabinosides.[329] The potential contribution of the prostaglandins to medicine is widely known and certain soft coral species produce some of these important substances. For example, subjecting the prostaglandin ester mixture from *Plexaura homomalla* to enzymatic hydrolysis has led to isolation of prostaglandins A_2, 5,6-*trans*-A_2, $F_{2\alpha}$, 13,14-*cis*-A_2, 13,14-dihydro-A acetate methyl ester, and the internal Michael adduct derived from 13,14-dihydro-A_2.[370] Interestingly, prostaglandin E_1 significantly inhibits growth of the B-16 melanoma cell line and a derivative 16-dimethyl-E_2 methyl ester significantly inhibits *in vivo* growth of this tumor system.[355] Useful amino acid derived marine animal medicinal agents range from the potent hypotensive undecapeptide eledoisin[19,326] (from the salivary gland of the octopus *Eledone moschata*) to the fish insulins. For example, preparations from tuna fish islets of Langerhan's were used to treat diabetic patients in Japan during the Second World War.[165]

Doubtlessly, a tremendous number of marine animal macromolecules will be discovered and found of utility in medicine. By way of illustration, we have isolated the first two antineoplastic agents from a shark (the hammerhead *Sphyrna lewini*) and both were found to be glycoproteins.[338] More recently we found two new glycoproteins in the green sea urchin, *Strongylocentrotus drobachiensis* that also significantly inhibit growth of the P388 murine lymphocytic leukemia.[336] At the time of writing we are in the process of uncovering several more antineoplastic proteins in relatively small marine vertebrates.[331] Quite likely the shark glycoproteins (sphyrnastatins 1 and 2) and other such protein antineoplastic substances act by stimulating the immune system to more effective measures against invading neoplastic disease. In this regard Sigel *et al.*[388] have been investigating serum proteins from the nurse shark *Ginglymostoma cirratum* in respect to immune antibody formation. On this basis, immunotherapy with crude macromolecular extracts such as BCG might better be considered as just another facet of cancer chemotherapy.

A good selection of marine animals from Florida and the Caribbean Island have been screened recently for cardiovasuclar and central nervous system active constituents and a number of promising leads were uncovered.[221a] Clearly the isolation of marine animal medicinal agents is only beginning. A contemporary synopsis of marine animal bio-organic chemistry can be obtained in reviews by Minale[293,294] of Porifera constituents, a treatment by Scheuer[360] of marine organism toxins, and in more comprehensive reviews.[26,137,138,140,361] The current thrust of marine animal natural products chemistry can be partially ascertained by considering the advances summarized from July to November 1977. Two new cembranolides from the soft coral *Sinularia flexibilis* were shown to be cytotoxic. The Weinheimer group[428] also found sinularin and dihydrosinularin to be accompanied by the known sinulariolide.[414] While no biological activity was described for any of the other new low molecular weight marine animal biosynthetic products, some of these structures suggest that such evaluation would be fruitful. For example, mycosporine from the Zoanthid *Palythoa tuberculosa* obtained by the Hirata group,[204] a new capnellene from the soft coral *Capnella imbricata* by the Djerassi and Tursch group,[383] the diterpene xenicin isolated by Schmitz and colleagues[423] from the soft coral

Sinularin
P388: ED$_{50}$, 0.3 μg/ml
KB: ED$_{50}$, 0.3 μg/ml
Reference 428

Dihydrosinularin
P388: ED$_{50}$, 20 μg/ml
KB: ED$_{50}$, 1.1 μg/ml
Reference 428

Sinulariolide
P388: ED$_{50}$, 7 μg/ml
KB: ED$_{50}$, 20 μg/ml
Reference 428

Mycosporine
Reference 204

Δ$^{9(12)}$-Capnellene-3β, 8β,10α,
14-tetrol
Reference 383

Xenicin
Reference 423

Zenia elongata, another unusual terpene (sester-)ircinianin (from a member of the sponge genus Ircinia in the Basel Laboratories of Hoffmann-LaRoche Laboratories),[185] our isolation of angasiol from the sea hare *Aplysia angasi,*[333] the pyrrolloterpene molliorin-B from the Italian sponge *Cacaspongia mollior,*[62] and the tryptophan derivative 6-bromohypaphorin

Ircinianin
Reference 185

Angasiol
Reference 333

Molliorin-B
Reference 62

from the British sponge *Pachymatisma johnstoni* by Thomson *et al.*[347] In the same period other sponge,[17,63] soft coral,[52,101] and sea hare[199,454]

6-Bromohypaphorine
Reference 347

terpenes were isolated. Five depsipeptides were isolated from the sea cucumber *Stichopus japonicus*,[200] three polypeptides with cardiotoxic and neurotoxic activity were obtained from the sea anemone *Anemonia sulcata*, and a toxin designated maculotoxin was isolated from the blue-ringed octopus *Hapalochlaena maculosa*.[107] A second toxin was obtained from the same octopus and called hapalotoxin,[356] On the basis of chromatographic behavior both of these posterior salivary gland components seemed related to tetrodotoxin and LD_{50} values of 50 and 150 μg/kg were found, respectively, for maculotoxin and hapalotoxin.[356] Understandably, the octopus *H. maculosa* has been responsible for a number of human deaths. Mosher and colleagues[322] have continued their investigation of Central American frogs for tetrodotoxin-like substances and have isolated the potent neurotoxins tetrodotoxin and chiriquitoxin from eggs of the Costa Rican *Atelopus chiriquiensis*. Since both toxins had to be extracted with 3% acetic acid and were not extracted by water it appears they might occur (in the eggs) in a bound form.

Several of the preceding new contributions to marine animal chemistry provide some striking illustrations of the abundance in which certain bio-synthetic products are produced, especially terpenes.[101,185,199,423] For example, 100 g of the crushed sponge *Ircinia sp.* was extracted with ligroin and upon concentrating and cooling 2.3 g of ircinianin crystallized.[185] Analogously, 100 g of a freeze-dried powder prepared from the soft coral *Sarcophyton sp.* when extracted with ligroin afforded upon concentration of the extract 0.3 g of a new cembrenoid diterpene.[101] However, the isola-tion of other types of compounds is generally more challenging than with higher plants and the discovery of antineoplastic constituents is usually considerably to exceedingly more difficult.

Primarily over the past twenty-five years a number of specialized isolatin techniques have been applied to marine animal problems. A selection of the more classic and workable approaches have been summarized in Schemes 1–6. The first two methods (Schemes 1, 2) have been employed to obtain a variety of hydrocarbons, long-chain alcohols, and sterols.[39,123] More recently the use of glc–mass spectrometry techniques with, for example, silyl ether derivatives has been developed, especially by Djerassi and colleagues,[112,302,303,341,342,378,381,400,420] into a most powerful technique for final purification and characterization of marine organism sterols. Scheme 3, developed by Scheuer and colleagues, has proved very effective for isolating sea urchin pigments.[308] The isolation of sea cucumber saponins has been of increasing interest due to their antifungal and cytotoxic properties[334] and Schemes 4 and 5 have been included to exemplify the earlier approach of Chanley[77] and the improved procedure of Djerassi.[350,379] The isolation of tetrodotoxin shown in Scheme 6 exemplifies an elegant separation procedure specifically designed for the isolation of tetrodotoxin in gram quantities.[161] By this means, 100 kg of chopped fresh ovaries from the puffer fish *Spheroides rubripes* in 200 liters of water led to 1–2 g yields of pure tetrodotoxin.[161]

For the past 12 years our group[337] has been exploring various separation techniques for isolating marine animal antineoplastic and/or cytotoxic constituents. The hitherto unpublished procedure outlined in Scheme 7 represents a generally workable approach for initial concentration of marine animal components for biological evaluation. In the 1965–1966 period one of us (GRP) began using 2-propanol routinely for preservation and shipment of field collections. Thus, removal of solvent from the 2-propanol solution serves as an initial extract. The residual marine animal or plant material is then treated as outlined in Scheme 7. Once the most promising fraction has been detected by bioassay, further separation is conducted using essentially all of the better known adsorption, gel permeation, ion exchange, and reverse phase chromatographic techniques outlined in Volume 2 of this series.[329] A great variety of other isolation methods effective for obtaining marine animal components can be obtained by consulting specific entries in Chapters 9–15.

As already noted in the preface, our need for the survey of data presented in the following chapters became acutely obvious about 1970. At the same time interest in marine animal chemistry began to increase markedly. In the next five years nearly 200 papers concerned with marine animal bio-organic chemistry appeared. This is in contrast to only 14 such manuscripts in the period 1900–1950, increasing to 34 in the 1950s and to 87 by the late 1960s. Consequently the data of Chapters 9–15 were prepared to provide ready access to information needed for the rapid identification of previously known constituents and to assist in characterization of new marine animal biosynthetic products. The data have been arranged according to the class of compound and each chapter has been sequenced on the basis of increasing empirical formula. When known with some certainty the structure has been entered along with a trivial name, if known; the melting point, optical rotation at the sodium-D line (with solvent), a notation concerning any spectral data, and the original marine organism have been noted. Biologically active fractions and other such mixtures were not included. Thus, only pure substances with reasonably well established structures are listed. Synthetic modifications of these marine animal natural products were not included unless they represented simple derivatives used for characterization. It is hoped that the data in the following chapters will encourage the investigation of many of these substances for biological activity. Only in a small number of instances does a biological study seem to have been initiated. Most of the substances listed have never been evaluated, for example, for antineoplastic and/or cytotoxic activity. The same observation applies to other areas of major medical interest.

SCHEME 1
Isolation of Hydrocarbons, Alcohols, and Sterols[39]

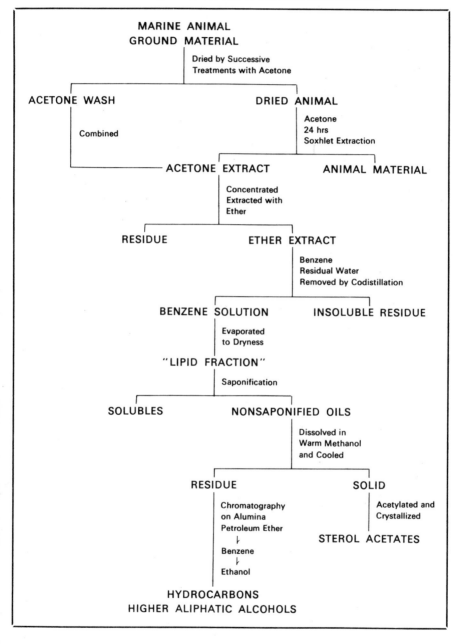

SCHEME 2
Isolation of Sterols[123]

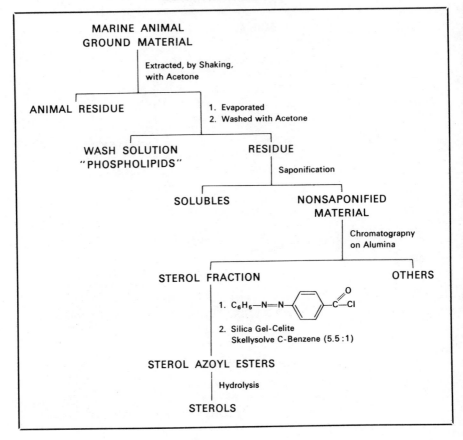

SCHEME 3
Separation of Pigments from Echinoids[308]

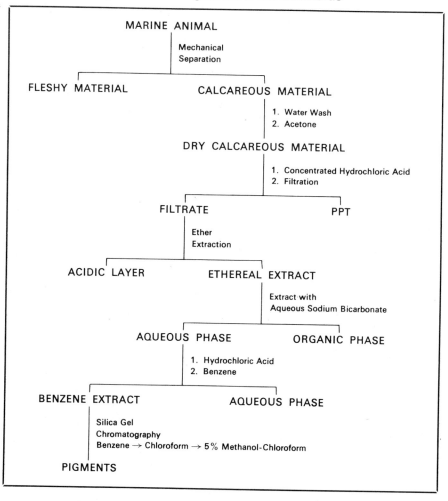

SCHEME 4
Isolation of Holothurins Method A[77]

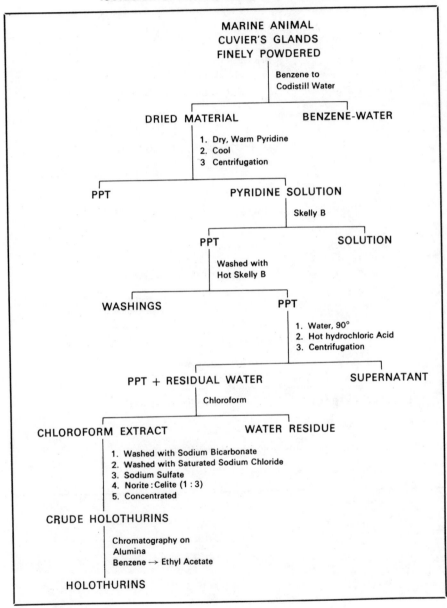

SCHEME 5
Isolation of Holothurins Method B[350]

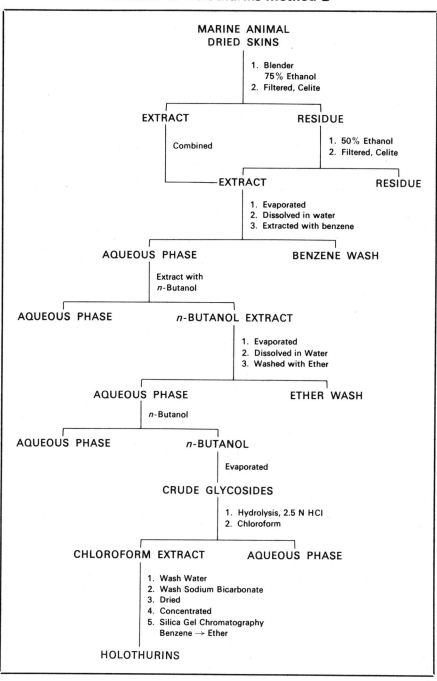

SCHEME 6
Separation of Tetrodotoxin[161]

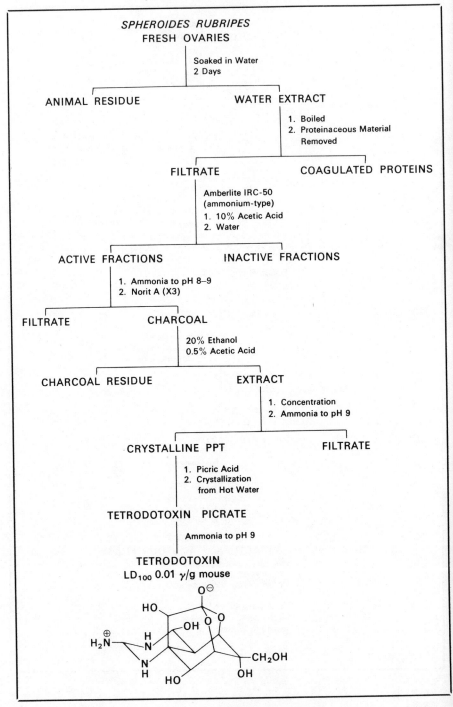

SPHEROIDES RUBRIPES
FRESH OVARIES

Soaked in Water
2 Days

ANIMAL RESIDUE   WATER EXTRACT

1. Boiled
2. Proteinaceous Material
   Removed

FILTRATE   COAGULATED PROTEINS

Amberlite IRC-50
(ammonium-type)
1. 10% Acetic Acid
2. Water

ACTIVE FRACTIONS   INACTIVE FRACTIONS

1. Ammonia to pH 8–9
2. Norit A (X3)

FILTRATE   CHARCOAL

20% Ethanol
0.5% Acetic Acid

CHARCOAL RESIDUE   EXTRACT

1. Concentration
2. Ammonia to pH 9

CRYSTALLINE PPT   FILTRATE

1. Picric Acid
2. Crystallization
   from Hot Water

TETRODOTOXIN PICRATE

Ammonia to pH 9

TETRODOTOXIN
LD_{100} 0.01 γ/g mouse

SCHEME 7
A Solvent Separation for Preliminary Biological Evaluation[337]

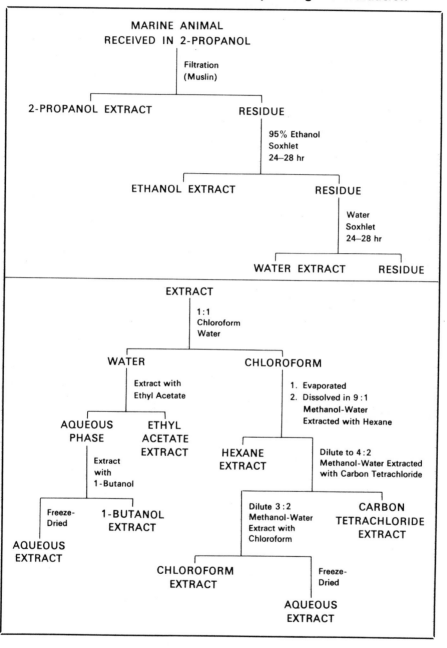

Chapter 9

Hydrocarbons, Alcohols, and Esters

C$_{14}$H$_{30}$O   **Tetradecanol**   CH$_3$(CH$_2$)$_{12}$CH$_2$OH

MOL. WT.: 214
MELTING POINT: 38–38.5°C; 3,5-Dinitrobenzoate, 66.5°C; Phenylurethane,
       70.5°C
ORGANISM: *Condylactis gigantea* (Coelenterata)
REFERENCE: 39

C$_{16}$H$_{16}$O   **Navenone B**

MOL. WT.: 224
MELTING POINT: 125–140°C
SPECTRAL DATA: UV, IR, PMR, Mass Spec
ORGANISM: *Navanax inermis* (Cooper) (Mollusca)
REFERENCE: 392

C$_{16}$H$_{16}$O$_2$ **Navenone C**

MOL. WT.: 240
MELTING POINT: Oil; Acetate 135–137°C
SPECTRAL DATA: UV, IR, PMR, Mass Spec
ORGANISM: *Navanax inermis* (Cooper) (Mollusca)
REFERENCE: 392

$C_{16}H_{34}O$ Hexadecanol $CH_3(CH_2)_{14}CH_2OH$

MOL. WT.: 242
MELTING POINT: 49°C; 3,5-Dinitrobenzoate, 72°C
ORGANISM: *Condylactis gigantea* (Coelenterata)
REFERENCE: 39

$C_{18}H_{38}O$ Octadecanol $CH_3(CH_2)_{16}CH_2OH$

MOL. WT.: 270
MELTING POINT: 56.5°C; Phenylurethane, 75.5°C
ORGANISM: *Condylactis gigantea* (Coelenterata)
REFERENCE: 39

$C_{22}H_{33}BrO$ Renierin-1

MOL. WT.: 394
MELTING POINT: Oil
SPECTRAL DATA: UV, IR, PMR, Mass Spec
ORGANISM: *Reniera fulva* (Porifera)
REFERENCE: 83

$C_{22}H_{34}O$ Debromorenierin-1

MOL. WT.: 314
MELTING POINT: Oil
SPECTRAL DATA: UV, IR, PMR, Mass Spec
ORGANISM: *Reniera fulva* (Porifera)
REFERENCE: 83

$C_{22}H_{35}BrO$ 18-Dihydrorenierin-1

MOL. WT.: 396
MELTING POINT: Oil
$[\alpha]_D$: −5.4   SOLVENT: Chf
SPECTRAL DATA: UV, IR, PMR, Mass Spec
ORGANISM: *Reniera fulva* (Porifera)
REFERENCE: 83

C$_{23}$H$_{38}$O   Renierin-2

MOL. WT.: 330
MELTING POINT: 35°C
SPECTRAL DATA: UV, IR, PMR, Mass Spec
ORGANISM: *Reniera fulva* (Porifera)
REFERENCE: 83

C$_{23}$H$_{38}$O$_2$ 18-Hydroxyrenierin-2

MOL. WT.: 346
MELTING POINT: 32°C
[α]$_D$: −38   SOLVENT: Me
SPECTRAL DATA: UV, IR, PMR, Mass Spec
ORGANISM: *Reniera fulva* (Porifera)
REFERENCE: 83

C$_{27}$H$_{56}$ Heptacosane

$$CH_3(CH_2)_{25}CH_3$$

MOL. WT.: 380
MELTING POINT: 59.5°C
ORGANISM: *Spheciospongia vesparia* (Porifera)
REFERENCE: 41

C$_{32}$H$_{64}$O$_2$ Cetyl palmitate

$$CH_3(CH_2)_{14}C\!\!-\!\!O(CH_2)_{15}CH_3$$
$$\overset{O}{\parallel}$$

MOL. WT.: 480
MELTING POINT: 50.9–51.5°C
ORGANISM: *Palythoa mammilosa* (Coelenterata)
REFERENCE: 39

Chapter 10

Sterols and Steroids

C₁₈H₂₄O₂   **Estradiol**

MOL. WT.: 272
MELTING POINT: 222°C
[α]ᴅ: +84
ORGANISM: *Torpedo marmorata* (Chordata/Pisces)
REFERENCE: 54

C₂₁H₃₂O₃

MOL. WT.: 332
MELTING POINT: 157–160°C
[α]ᴅ: +65.2
SPECTRAL DATA: IR, PMR, Mass Spec
ORGANISM: *Asterias amurensis* Lutkin
    (Echinodermata)
REFERENCE: 198, 455

C₂₁H₃₂O₆S

MOL. WT.: 412
MELTING POINT: 160–161°C
[α]ᴅ: +20
SPECTRAL DATA: PMR
ORGANISM: *Asterias amurensis* Lutkin
    (Echinodermata)
REFERENCE: 196

C₂₅H₃₈O

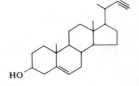

MOL. WT.: 354
MELTING POINT: 104–105°C; Acetate, 122–125°C
[α]_D: −42.2
SPECTRAL DATA: IR, PMR, Mass Spec
ORGANISM: *Calyx nicaaensis* (Porifera)
REFERENCE: 400

C₂₆H₄₀O

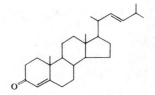

MOL. WT.: 368
SPECTRAL DATA: PMR, Mass Spec
ORGANISM: *Stelleta clarella* (Porifera)
REFERENCE: 381

C₂₆H₄₂O   Asterosterol

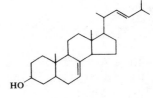

MOL. WT.: 370
MELTING POINT: 129–130°C; Acetate, 134–135°C
[α]_D: 0
SPECTRAL DATA: IR, Mass Spec
ORGANISM: *Asterias amurensis* Lutkin
           (Echinodermata)
REFERENCE: 247

C₂₆H₄₂O

MOL. WT. 370
MELTING POINT: 137–138°C; Acetate, 131–132.5°C;
               Propionate, 113–115°C
SPECTRAL DATA: PMR, Mass Spec
ORGANISM: *Cliona celata, Stelleta clarella, Tethya
           aurantia, Lissodendoryx noxiosa, Haliclona
           permollis,* and *Haliclona* sp. (Porifera)
REFERENCE: 119, 381

$C_{26}H_{42}O$

MOL. WT.: 370
MELTING POINT: 104–105°C
$[\alpha]_D$: −52
SPECTRAL DATA: IR, PMR, Mass Spec
ORGANISM: *Placopecten magellanicus* Gmelin
           (Mollusca)
REFERENCE: 194

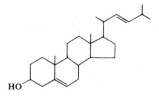

$C_{26}H_{42}O$

MOL. WT.: 370
MELTING POINT: 143–144°C; Acetate, 142.5–143°C
$[\alpha]_D$: −65
ORGANISM: *Placopecten magellanicus* Gmelin
           (Mollusca)
REFERENCE: 148, 149

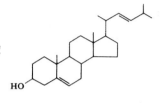

$C_{26}H_{44}O$

MOL. WT.: 372
MELTING POINT: Acetate, 103–105°C
ORGANISM: *Axinella polypoides* (Porifera)
REFERENCE: 299

$C_{26}H_{44}O$

MOL. WT. 372
MELTING POINT: 85°C; 119–121°C; Acetate,
           116–121°C
ORGANISM: *Hymeniacidon perleve* (Porifera)
REFERENCE: 119

$C_{27}H_{40}O_4$

MOL. WT.: 428
MELTING POINT: 151–151.5°C
SPECTRAL DATA: UV, IR, PMR, Mass Spec
ORGANISM: *Ptilosarcus gurneyi* (Gray)
           (Coelenterata)
REFERENCE: 420

C₂₇H₄₂O

MOL. WT.:   382
SPECTRAL DATA: Mass Spec
ORGANISM: *Stelleta clarella* (Porifera)
REFERENCE: 381

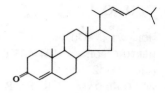

C₂₇H₄₂O

MOL. WT.:   382
MELTING POINT: 119–120°C; Acetate, 151–153°C
[α]ᴅ: −38.8
SPECTRAL DATA: IR, PMR, Mass Spec
ORGANISM: *Calyx nicaaensis* (Porifera)
REFERENCE: 400

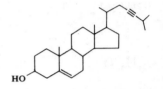

C₂₇H₄₂O₂

MOL. WT.:   398
MELTING POINT: 138–140°C
[α]ᴅ: +43.2   SOLVENT: Chf
SPECTRAL DATA: IR, PMR, Mass Spec
ORGANISM: *Acanthaster planci* Linn.
             (Echinodermata)
REFERENCE: 386

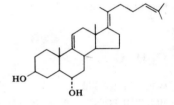

C₂₇H₄₂O₃

MOL. WT.:   414
MELTING POINT: 202–206°C; Acetate, 147–150°C
[α]ᴅ: −17.5   SOLVENT: Chf
SPECTRAL DATA: PMR, Mass Spec
ORGANISM: *Axinella cannabina* (Porifera)
REFERENCE: 130

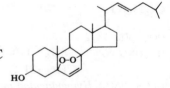

C₂₇H₄₂O₃

MOL. WT.:   414
ORGANISM: *Marthasterias glacialis*
             (Echinodermata)
REFERENCE: 394

$C_{27}H_{44}O$ Amuresterol

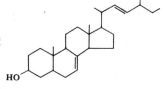

MOL. WT.: 384
MELTING POINT: 151–153°C; Acetate, 161–163°C
$[\alpha]_D$: +3
SPECTRAL DATA: IR, PMR, Mass Spec
ORGANISM: *Asterias amurensis* Lutkin
          (Echinodermata)
REFERENCE: 245

$C_{27}H_{44}O$

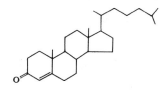

MOL. WT.: 384
SPECTRAL DATA: Mass Spec
ORGANISM: *Stelleta clarella* (Porifera)
REFERENCE: 381

$C_{27}H_{44}O$

MOL. WT.: 384
MELTING POINT: 134–136°C; Acetate, 128–131°C;
                 4-Bromoacetate, 178–179°C
$[\alpha]_D$: −58.5   SOLVENT: Chf
SPECTRAL DATA: IR
ORGANISM: *Placopecten magellanicus* Gmelin
          (Mollusca), *Stelleta clarella*, *Tethya aurantia*, and *Lissodendoryx*
          noxiosa (Porifera)
REFERENCE: 381, 407, 456

$C_{27}H_{44}O$

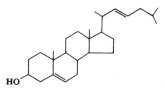

MOL. WT.: 384
MELTING POINT: Acetate, 129–130°C
$[\alpha]_D$: −19.2   SOLVENT: Chf
ORGANISM: *Stelleta clarella*, *Tethya aurantia*,
          and *Lissodendoryx noxiosa*
          (Porifera)
REFERENCE: 381

C₂₇H₄₄O

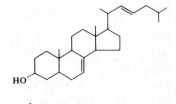

MOL. WT.: 384
MELTING POINT: 129–130.5°C; Acetate,
140–142.5°C
[α]ᴅ: −4.2   SOLVENT: Chf
SPECTRAL DATA: IR, Mass Spec
ORGANISM: *Asterias amurensis* Lutkin (Echinodermata)
REFERENCE: 247

C₂₇H₄₄O

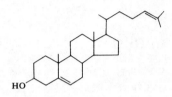

MOL. WT.: 384
MELTING POINT: 117°C; Acetate, 101.5°C;
Benzoate, 129°C
[α]ᴅ: −38.7   SOLVENT: Chf
ORGANISM: *Balanus glandula* (Arthropoda/Crustacea)
REFERENCE: 124

C₂₇H₄₄O

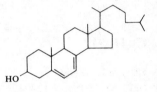

MOL. WT.: 384
MELTING POINT: Acetate, 176.5°C
ORGANISM: *Madrepora cervicornis* (Coelenterata)
REFERENCE: 42

C₂₇H₄₄O

MOL. WT.: 384
MELTING POINT: 128.5–129.5°C; Acetate, 138–141°C
[α]ᴅ: −43
SPECTRAL DATA: IR, PMR, Mass Spec
ORGANISM: *Pseudopotamilla occelata* Moore
(Annelida)
REFERENCE: 244

C₂₇H₄₄O₃

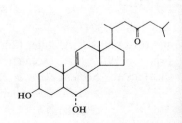

MOL. WT.: 416
MELTING POINT: 167–169°C
SPECTRAL DATA: IR, PMR, Mass Spec
ORGANISM: *Marthasterias glacialis*
(Echinodermata)
REFERENCE: 394

$C_{27}H_{44}O_4$ Thornasterol A

MOL. WT.: 432

MELTING POINT: Diacetate, 158–159°C

ORGANISM: *Acanthaster planci* Linn.
(Echinodermata)

REFERENCE: 236

$C_{27}H_{44}O_6$ 2-Deoxycrustecdysone

MOL. WT.: 464

SPECTRAL DATA: IR, PMR, Mass Spec

ORGANISM: *Jasus lalandei* (Chordata/Pisces)

REFERENCE: 156, 157

$C_{27}H_{44}O_7$ Callinecdysone A

MOL. WT.: 480

ORGANISM: *Callinectes sapidus* (Arthropoda/Curstacea)

REFERENCE: 143

$C_{27}H_{44}O_7$ Crustecdysone

MOL. WT.: 480

MELTING POINT: 150–151°C

SPECTRAL DATA: UV, IR, PMR, Mass Spec

ORGANISM: *Jasus lalandei* (Chordata/Pisces),
Polypodium vulgare L. (Coelenterata), and *Callinectes sapidus*
(Arthropoda/Crustacea)

REFERENCE: 143, 172, 187, 188, 206

$C_{27}H_{46}O$ Cholesterol

MOL. WT.: 386
MELTING POINT: 148°C; Acetate, 116°
$[\alpha]_D$: -40.2 SOLVENT: Chf
SPECTRAL DATA: Mass Spec
ORGANISM: *Balanus glandula, Chionoecetes opilio, Paralithodes* sp. (Arthropoda/
Crustacea), *Zoanthus confertus* (Coelenterata), *Ctenodiseus
crispatus* Retzius, *Asterina pectinifera, Asterias amurensis* Lutkin,
*Distolasterias sticantha, Certonardoa semiregularis, Lysastrosoma
anthostictha, Solaster paxillatas* (Echinodermata), *Muricea
appressa, Plexaura* sp., *Eugorgia ampla* (Coelenterata), *Artemia
salina* L. (Arthropoda/Crustaceae), *Meandra areolata*
(Coelenterata), *Suberites compacta* (Porifera), *Pseudopotamilla
occelata* Moore (Annelida), *Cliona celata, Hymeniacidon perleve*
(Porifera), *Lytechinus variegatus* (Echinodermata), and *Axinella
cannabina* (Porifera)
REFERENCE: 40, 42, 47, 64, 81, 119, 124, 166, 167, 168, 193, 246, 248, 253,
323, 456

$C_{27}H_{46}O$ Lathosterol

MOL. WT.: 386
MELTING POINT: 121–123°C; Acetate,
116–118°C;
153–155°C
$[\alpha]_D$: $+4.3$
ORGANISM: *Chiton tuberculatus* L. (Mollusca)
REFERENCE: 230

$C_{27}H_{46}O$

MOL. WT.: 386
MELTING POINT: Acetate, 112–113°C
ORGANISM: *Axinella polypoides* (Porifera)
REFERENCE: 299

$C_{27}H_{46}O_3$

MOL. WT.: 418
MELTING POINT: 240–243°C
$[\alpha]_D$: $+41.5$ SOLVENT: EtOH
SPECTRAL DATA: Mass Spec
ORGANISM: *Asterias amurensis* Lutkin
(Echinodermata)
REFERENCE: 197

$C_{27}H_{46}O_5$ **Scymanol**

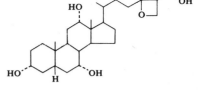

MOL. WT.: 450
MELTING POINT: 186–188°C; Tetra-acetate
          145.5–147°C
ORGANISM: *Galeocerdo arcticus*, and
          Scymnus borealis
          (Chordata/Pisces)
REFERENCE: 44, 108

$C_{27}H_{48}O$ **Cholestanol**

MOL. WT.: 388
MELTING POINT: 142°C
$[\alpha]_D$: +24   SOLVENT: Chf
SPECTRAL DATA: PMR, Mass Spec
ORGANISM: *Stelleta clarella, Tethya aurantia, Lissodendoryx noxiosa*, and
          Haliclona sp. (Porifera)
REFERENCE: 381

$C_{27}H_{48}O$

MOL. WT.: 388
MELTING POINT: Acetate, 64–65°C
ORGANISM: *Axinella verrucosa* (Porifera)
REFERENCE: 298

$C_{27}H_{48}O_4$

MOL. WT.: 436
MELTING POINT: 197–199.5°C; per Acetate, 137–138°C
$[\alpha]_D$: +45.7   SOLVENT: Me
SPECTRAL DATA: IR, PMR, Mass Spec
ORGANISM: *Asterias amurensis* Lutkin
          (Echinodermata)
REFERENCE: 211

$C_{28}H_{44}O$

MOL. WT.: 396
SPECTRAL DATA: Mass Spec
ORGANISM: *Stelleta clarella* (Porifera)
REFERENCE: 381

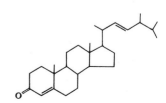

C₂₈H₄₄O

$C_{28}H_{44}O$

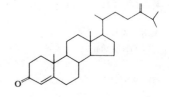

MOL. WT.: 396
MELTING POINT: 115°C
[α]_D: +89.1   SOLVENT: Chf
SPECTRAL DATA: PMR, Mass Spec
ORGANISM: *Stelleta clarella* (Porifera)
REFERENCE: 381

$C_{28}H_{44}O_3$

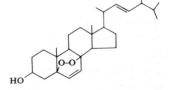

MOL. WT.: 428
MELTING POINT: 180–184°C; Acetate, 196–199°C
SPECTRAL DATA: IR, PMR, Mass Spec
ORGANISM: *Axinella cannabina* (Porifera)
REFERENCE: 130

$C_{28}H_{46}O$ Episterol

MOL. WT.: 398
MELTING POINT: 131°C; Acetate, 140°C; Benzoate,
          160°C
[α]_D: +6.0   SOLVENT: Chf
SPECTRAL DATA: IR, PMR
ORGANISM: *Pisaster ochraceus*, and *Asterias
          amurensis* Lutkin (Echinodermata)
REFERENCE: 43, 123, 254

$C_{28}H_{46}O$ Brassicasterol, Chondrillastanol,
          Poriferastanol

MOL. WT.: 398
MELTING POINT: 157–158°C; Acetate, 139–140°C;
          Benzoate, 111°C
[α]_D: −39.4   SOLVENT: Chf
SPECTRAL DATA: Mass Spec
ORGANISM: *Stelleta clarella, Tethya aurantia, Lissodendoryx noxiosa, Haliclona
          permollis, Haliclona* sp., and *Chondrilla nucula* Schmidt (Porifera)
REFERENCE: 43, 381

C$_{28}$H$_{46}$O

MOL. WT.: 398
MELTING POINT: 140–142°C; Acetate, 132–134°C;
Benzoate, 148°C
[α]$_D$: −3.95   SOLVENT: Chf
SPECTRAL DATA: IR, Mass Spec
ORGANISM: *Stelleta clarella, Tethya aurantia,*
Lissodendoryx noxiosa, Haliclona permollis, Haliclona sp.
(Porifera), *Palythoa* sp. (Coelenterata), *Saxidomus giganteus,*
Pecten caurinus, Cardium corbis, Modiolus demissus (Mollusca)
REFERENCE: 125, 167, 192, 381

C$_{28}$H$_{46}$O   Stellasterol

MOL. WT.: 398
MELTING POINT: 159–161°C; Acetate, 181–182°C
[α]$_D$: +7.8   SOLVENT: Chf
ORGANISM: *Asterias amurensis* Lutkin
(Echinodermata)
REFERENCE: 247

C$_{28}$H$_{46}$O$_2$ Callinecdysone B

MOL. WT.: 494
ORGANISM: *Callinectes sapidus* (Arthropoda/
Crustacea)
REFERENCE: 143

C$_{28}$H$_{46}$O$_2$

MOL. WT.: 414
ORGANISM: *Acanthaster planci* Linn.
(Echinodermata)
REFERENCE: 386

C$_{28}$H$_{46}$O$_2$

MOL. WT.: 414
SPECTRAL DATA: Mass Spec
ORGANISM: *Pseudoplexaura porosa* (Coelenterata)
REFERENCE: 342

$C_{28}H_{46}O_3$ 24-Methylenecholest-5-en-3β,7β,19-triol

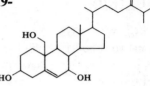

MOL. WT.:   430
MELTING POINT: 112–114°C
$[\alpha]_D$:   +16   SOLVENT: Me
SPECTRAL DATA: IR, PMR, Mass Spec
ORGANISM: *Litophyton viridis* (Coelenterata)
REFERENCE: 50

$C_{28}H_{46}O_4$ Thornasterol B

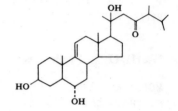

MOL. WT.:   446
MELTING POINT: Diacetate, 147–148°C
ORGANISM: *Acanthaster planci* Linn.
                (Echinodermata)
REFERENCE: 236

$C_{28}H_{48}O$ Campesterol

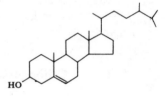

MOL. WT.:   400
MELTING POINT: 158°C; Acetate, 138°C;
                3,5-Dinitrobenzoate, 203°C
$[\alpha]_D$:   −33
SPECTRAL DATA: Mass Spec
ORGANISM: *Stelleta clarella*, and *Tethya aurantia*
                (Porifera)
REFERENCE: 144, 381

$C_{28}H_{48}O$ Neospongosterol

MOL. WT.:   400
MELTING POINT: 153°C; Acetate, 141–142°C;
                Benzoate, 146°C
$[\alpha]_D$:   +10
ORGANISM: *Suberites compacta* (Porifera)
REFERENCE: 40

$C_{28}H_{48}O$

MOL. WT.:   400
MELTING POINT: Acetate, 116–117°C
ORGANISM: *Axinella polypoides* (Porifera)
REFERENCE: 299

$C_{28}H_{48}O$

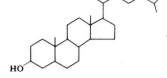

MOL. WT.: 400
MELTING POINT: 110–115°C; Acetate, 123–125°C
ORGANISM: *Hymeniacidon perleve* (Porifera)
REFERENCE: 119

$C_{28}H_{48}O_2$

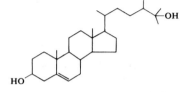

MOL. WT.: 416
MELTING POINT: 189.5–190.5°C; Acetate,
151–152°C
$[\alpha]_D$: -47.1
SPECTRAL DATA: IR, PMR, Mass Spec
ORGANISM: *Alcyonarian nephtea* (Coelenterata)
REFERENCE: 117

$C_{28}H_{50}O$

MOL. WT.: 402
MELTING POINT: Acetate, 84–86°C
SPECTRAL DATA: PMR, Mass Spec
ORGANISM: *Axinella verrucosa* (Porifera)
REFERENCE: 298

CH₂OH

$C_{29}H_{44}O_6$ Heteronemin

MOL. WT.: 488
MELTING POINT: 176.5–177°
SPECTRAL DATA: PMR, Mass Spec
ORGANISM: *Heteronema erecta* (Porifera)
REFERENCE: 224

OAc
OH
O
OAc

$C_{29}H_{46}O$ Calysterol

MOL. WT.: 410
MELTING POINT: 114–116°C; Acetate, 104–106°C
$[\alpha]_D$: -29.3
SPECTRAL DATA: IR, PMR, Mass Spec
ORGANISM: *Calyx nicaensis* (Porifera)
REFERENCE: 127

HO

C$_{29}$H$_{46}$O

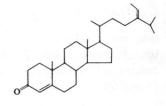

MOL. WT.: 410
MELTING POINT: 94–95°C
[α]$_D$: +80   SOLVENT: Chf
SPECTRAL DATA: PMR, Mass Spec
ORGANISM: *Stelleta clarella* (Porifera)
REFERENCE: 381

C$_{29}$H$_{48}$O   Chondrillasterol

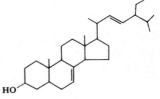

MOL. WT.: 412
MELTING POINT: 168–169°C; Acetate, 175–176°C;
              Benzoate, 194–195°C
[α]$_D$: −1.1
ORGANISM: *Chondrilla nucula* Schmidt (Porifera)
REFERENCE: 43

C$_{29}$H$_{48}$O   23-Demethyl-gorgosterol

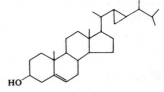

MOL. WT.: 412
MELTING POINT: 162–163°C
[α]$_D$: −34.5
SPECTRAL DATA: PMR, Mass Spec
ORGANISM: *Gorgonia flabellum* L., and *Gorgonia
          ventibna* L. (Coelenterata)
REFERENCE: 118, 367

C$_{29}$H$_{48}$O

MOL. WT.: 412
SPECTRAL DATA: PMR, Mass Spec
ORGANISM: *Stelleta clarella, Tethya aurantia,
          Lissodendoryx noxiosa, Haliclona
          permollis,* and *Haliclona* sp.
          (Porifera)
REFERENCE: 381

C₂₉H₄₈O

MOL. WT.: 412
MELTING POINT: 124°C
[α]ᴅ: −41.2   SOLVENT: Chf
SPECTRAL DATA: Mass Spec
ORGANISM: *Stelleta clarella, Tethya aurantia,*
　　　　　　Lissodendoryx noxiosa, Haliclona permollis,
　　　　　　and *Haliclona* sp. (Porifera)
REFERENCE: 381

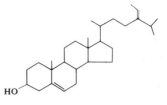

C₂₉H₄₈O　　24,28-Didehydroaplysterol dsp-1

MOL. WT.: 412
MELTING POINT: 128–130°C; Acetate, 113–114°C
[α]ᴅ: −37   SOLVENT: Cte
SPECTRAL DATA: IR, PMR, Mass Spec
ORGANISM: *Aplysina* (or *Verongia*) *aerophoba*
　　　　　　(Porifera)
REFERENCE: 110

C₂₉H₄₈O

MOL. WT.: 412
MELTING POINT: 127–129°C
SPECTRAL DATA: Mass Spec
ORGANISM: *Stelleta clarella, Tethya aurantia,*
　　　　　　Lissodendoryx noxiosa, Haliclona
　　　　　　permollis, and *Haliclona* sp. (Porifera)
REFERENCE: 381

C₂₉H₄₈O₂

MOL. WT.: 428
SPECTRAL DATA: Mass Spec
ORGANISM: *Pseudoplexaura porosa* (Coelenterata)
REFERENCE: 342

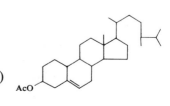

C₂₉H₅₀O   Aplysterol

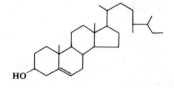

MOL. WT.: 414
MELTING POINT: 135–136°C; Acetate, 119–120°
[α]ᴅ: −25   SOLVENT: Chf
SPECTRAL DATA: PMR, Mass Spec
ORGANISM: *Aplysina* (or *Verongia*) *aerophoba*
          (Porifera)
REFERENCE: 110

C₂₉H₅₀O   β-Sitosterol

MOL. WT.: 414
MELTING POINT: 132°C
[α]ᴅ: −38.7
ORGANISM: *Verongia fistularis* (Porifera)
REFERENCE: 374, 377

C₂₉H₅₀O

MOL. WT.: 414
ORGANISM: *Periphylla periphylla* (Coelenterata)
REFERENCE: 28

C₂₉H₅₀O   Clionasterol

MOL. WT.: 414
MELTING POINT: 136°C; Propionate, 114–115°C;
          Acetate, 140–141°C;
          3,5-Dinitrobenzoate, 202°C
[α]ᴅ: −34
SPECTRAL DATA: PMR, Mass Spec
ORGANISM: *Stelleta clarella, Lissodendoryx noxiosa* (Porifera),
          and *Xiphogergia* sp. (Coelenterata)
REFERENCE: 42, 153, 381

$C_{29}H_{52}O$

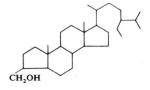

MOL. WT.:   416
MELTING POINT: Acetate, 86–88°C
ORGANISM: *Axinella verrucosa* (Porifera)
REFERENCE: 298

$C_{30}H_{46}O_4$

MOL. WT.:   470
MELTING POINT: 202–203°C
$[\alpha]_D$:   +10.5   SOLVENT: Chf
SPECTRAL DATA: UV, IR, PMR, Mass Spec
ORGANISM: *Thelonota ananas* Jaeger (Echinodermata)
REFERENCE: 225

$C_{30}H_{48}O_2$

MOL. WT.:   440
ORGANISM: *Pseudoplexaura porosa* (Coelenterata)
REFERENCE: 342

$C_{30}H_{48}O_4$

MOL. WT.:   472
MELTING POINT: 229–232°C
$[\alpha]_D$:   +6.2   SOLVENT: Chf
SPECTRAL DATA: UV, IR, PMR, Mass Spec
ORGANISM: *Thelonota ananas* Jaeger (Echinodermata)
REFERENCE: 225

$C_{30}H_{48}O_4$

MOL. WT.:   472
MELTING POINT: Amorphous
$[\alpha]_D$:   +53   SOLVENT: Me
SPECTRAL DATA: IR, PMR, Mass Spec
ORGANISM: *Litophyton viridis* (Coelenterata)
REFERENCE: 50

C$_{30}$H$_{48}$O$_5$

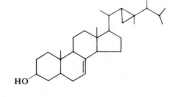

MOL. WT.: 488
MELTING POINT: 227–228°C
[α]$_D$: −1.3   SOLVENT: Chf
SPECTRAL DATA: UV, IR, PMR, Mass Spec
ORGANISM: *Thelonota ananas* Jaeger (Echinodermata)
REFERENCE: 225

C$_{30}$H$_{50}$O   Acanthasterol

MOL. WT.: 426
MELTING POINT: 179–180°C; *p*-Bromobenzoate, 230–232°C;
                    p-Iodobenzoate, 219–221°C
[α]$_D$: +5   SOLVENT: Chf
SPECTRAL DATA: IR, PMR, Mass Spec
ORGANISM: *Acanthaster planci* Linn. (Echinodermata)
REFERENCE: 168, 384, 385

C$_{30}$H$_{50}$O   Gorgastanone

MOL. WT.: 426
MELTING POINT: 203–206°C
SPECTRAL DATA: Mass Spec
REFERENCE: 171

C$_{30}$H$_{50}$O   Gorgosterol

MOL. WT.: 426
MELTING POINT: 186.5–188°C; Dihydro,
                    188.5–192°C; 3β-Bromo,
                    159–160°C
[α]$_D$: −45
SPECTRAL DATA: PMR, Mass Spec
ORGANISM: *Palythoa tuberculara* (Coelenterata)
REFERENCE: 167, 171, 280

$C_{30}H_{50}O$

MOL. WT.: 426
SPECTRAL DATA: Mass Spec
ORGANISM: *Tethya aurantia* (Porifera)
REFERENCE: 381

$C_{30}H_{52}$ **Gorgostane**

MOL. WT.: 412
MELTING POINT: 142–144°C
SPECTRAL DATA: Mass Spec
REFERENCE: 171

$C_{30}H_{52}O_5$

MOL. WT.: 492
MELTING POINT: 233–236°C
$[\alpha]_D$: −11   SOLVENT: Alc
SPECTRAL DATA: IR, PMR, Mass Spec
ORGANISM: *Sarcophyton elegans* Moser
      (Coelenterata)
REFERENCE: 303

$C_{30}H_{52}O_6$

MOL. WT.: 508
MELTING POINT: 248–255°C (dec.)
$[\alpha]_D$: −9.4   SOLVENT: Me
SPECTRAL DATA: PMR, Mass Spec
ORGANISM: *Sarcophyton elegans* Moser
      (Coelenterata)
REFERENCE: 302

$C_{31}H_{52}O_4$

MOL. WT.: 488
ORGANISM: *Pseudopterogorgia americana* Gmelin
      (Coelenterata)
REFERENCE: 118

C$_{32}$H$_{48}$O$_5$

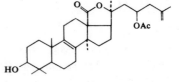

MOL. WT.: 512
MELTING POINT: 196–198°C
SPECTRAL DATA: UV, IR, PMR, Mass Spec
ORGANISM: *Thelonota ananas* Jaeger
            (Echinodermata)
REFERENCE: 226

C$_{32}$H$_{48}$O$_5$

MOL. WT.: 512
MELTING POINT: 225–227°C
[α]$_D$: −4   SOLVENT: Chf
SPECTRAL DATA: UV, IR, PMR, Mass Spec
ORGANISM: *Thelonota ananas* Jaeger (Echinodermata)
REFERENCE: 225

C$_{32}$H$_{50}$O$_5$

MOL. WT.: 514
MELTING POINT: 198–201°C
[α]$_D$: +13.8   SOLVENT: Me
SPECTRAL DATA: UV, IR, PMR, Mass Spec
ORGANISM: *Thelonota ananas* Jaeger (Echinodermata)
REFERENCE: 226

C$_{32}$H$_{50}$O$_5$

MOL. WT.: 514
MELTING POINT: 221–222°C
[α]$_D$: −18   SOLVENT: Chf
SPECTRAL DATA: UV, IR, PMR, Mass Spec
ORGANISM: *Thelonota ananas* Jaeger (Echinodermata)
REFERENCE: 225

$C_{32}H_{50}O_6$

MOL. WT.: 530
MELTING POINT: 203–205°C
$[\alpha]_D$: −10   SOLVENT: Chf
SPECTRAL DATA: UV, IR, PMR, Mass Spec
ORGANISM: *Thelonota ananas* Jaeger (Echinodermata)
REFERENCE: 225

$C_{33}H_{44}O_7$

MOL. WT.: 551
MELTING POINT: 127–130°C; Tetraacetate,
                 222–224°C
$[\alpha]_D$: −9.0   SOLVENT: Chf
SPECTRAL DATA: Mass Spec
ORGANISM: *Acanthaster planci* Linn.
              (Echinodermata)
REFERENCE: 382

$C_{50}H_{80}O_{24}$ dsp-1

MOL. WT.: 1064
MELTING POINT: 264–265°C
$[\alpha]_D$: +22   SOLVENT: Aq Me
SPECTRAL DATA: IR
ORGANISM: *Acanthaster planci* Linn.
              (Echinodermata)
REFERENCE: 235

Chapter 11

Terpenoids

$C_9H_8Br_2O_4$ Aeroplysinin-2

MOL. WT.: 340
MELTING POINT: 127–128°C
$[\alpha]_D$: +22   SOLVENT: MeOH
SPECTRAL DATA: UV, IR, PMR
ORGANISM: *Aplysina* (or *Verongia*) *aerophoba*, and
              Ianthella sp. (Porifera)
REFERENCE: 300

$C_{10}H_{12}Br_3Cl_3$

MOL. WT.: 478
MELTING POINT: 54°C
$[\alpha]_D$: −50.2
SPECTRAL DATA: PMR, Mass Spec
ORGANISM: *Aplysia californica* (Mollusca)
REFERENCE: 141

$C_{14}H_9Br_3O_3$ Thelepin

MOL. WT.: 465
MELTING POINT: 202–203°C (dec.); Acetate, 190°C
SPECTRAL DATA: UV, IR, PMR, Mass Spec
ORGANISM: *Thelepus setosus* (Annelida)
REFERENCE: 179, 180

$C_{14}H_{11}Br_3O_3$ Thelephenol

MOL. WT.: 467
MELTING POINT: 183–184°C
ORGANISM: *Thelepus setosus* (Annelida)
REFERENCE: 179, 180

$C_{14}H_{18}O_3$ Gyrinal

MOL. WT.: 234
SPECTRAL DATA: UV, PMR, Mass Spec
ORGANISM: *Gyrinidae* (Arthropoda/Insecta)
REFERENCE: 362

$C_{15}H_{16}O$ Pallescensin E

MOL. WT.: 212
MELTING POINT: oil
SPECTRAL DATA: UV, PMR, Mass Spec
ORGANISM: *Disidea pallescens* (Porifera)
REFERENCE: 86

$C_{15}H_{16}O$ Spiniferin-1

MOL. WT.: 212
MELTING POINT: Oil
$[\alpha]_D$: −4.2
SPECTRAL DATA: UV, PMR, Mass Spec
ORGANISM: *Pleraplysilla spinifera* (Porifera)
REFERENCE: 98

$C_{15}H_{16}O$ Spiniferin-2

MOL. WT.: 212
MELTING POINT: Oil
$[\alpha]_D$: 0
SPECTRAL DATA: UV, PMR, Mass Spec
ORGANISM: *Pleraplysilla spinifera* (Porifera)
REFERENCE: 98

C$_{15}$H$_{18}$O   **Furvoventalene**

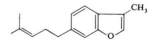

MOL. WT.: 214
METLING POINT: Liquid
SPECTRAL DATA: UV, PMR, Mass Spec
ORGANISM: *Gorgonia ventalina* (Coelenterata)
REFERENCE: 433

C$_{15}$H$_{18}$O   **Pallescensin C**

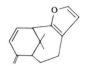

MOL. WT.: 214
MELTING POINT: Oil
[α]$_D$: +424
SPECTRAL DATA: UV, IR, Mass Spec
ORGANISM: *Disidea pallescens* (Porifera)
REFERENCE: 85

C$_{15}$H$_{18}$O   **Pallescensin D**

MOL. WT.: 214
MELTING POINT: Oil
[α]$_D$: −45.3
SPECTRAL DATA: UV, IR, PMR, Mass Spec
ORGANISM: *Disidea pallescens* (Porifera)
REFERENCE: 85

C$_{15}$H$_{18}$O   **Pallescensin F**

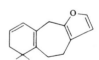

MOL. WT.: 214
MELTING POINT: Oil
SPECTRAL DATA: UV, PMR, Mass Spec
ORGANISM: *Disidea pallescens* (Porifera)
REFERENCE: 86

C$_{15}$H$_{18}$O   **Pallescensin G**

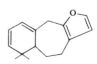

MOL. WT.: 214
MELTING POINT: Oil
[α_D]: −289
SPECTRAL DATA: UV, PMR, Mass Spec
ORGANISM: *Disidea pallescens* (Porifera)
REFERENCE: 86

$C_{15}H_{18}O_2$ **Longifolin**

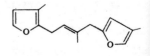

MOL. WT.: 230
ORGANISM: *Pleraplysilla spinifera* (Porifera)
REFERENCE: 98

$C_{15}H_{18}O_3$

MOL. WT.: 246
MELTING POINT: 99–100°C
$[\alpha]_D$: 0
SPECTRAL DATA: UV, IR, PMR, Mass Spec
ORGANISM: *Sinularia gonatodes* (Coelenterata)
REFERENCE: 102

$C_{15}H_{19}BrO$ **Aplysin**

MOL. WT.: 295
MELTING POINT: 85–86°C
$[\alpha]_D$: −85.4
SPECTRAL DATA: UV, IR, PMR, Mass Spec
ORGANISM: *Aplysia kurodai* (Mollusca)
REFERENCE: 453

$C_{15}H_{19}BrO_2$ **Aplysinol**

MOL. WT.: 311
MELTING POINT: 158–160°C
$[\alpha]_D$: −55.6
SPECTAL DATA: UV, IR, PMR,
ORGANISM: *Aplysia kurodai* (Mollusca)
REFERENCE: 453

$C_{15}H_{19}Br_2ClO$ **Dactylene**

MOL. WT.: 411
MELTING POINT: 62–63°C
$[\alpha]_D$: −36   SOLVENT: Chf
SPECTRAL DATA: UV, IR, PMR, Mass Spec
ORGANISM: *Aplysia dactylomela* (Mollusca)
REFERENCE: 291

$C_{15}H_{19}Br_2ClO$ Isodactylyne

MOL. WT.: 412
MELTING POINT: Oil
$[\alpha]_D$: -8.06 SOLVENT: Chf
SPECTRAL DATA: UV, IR, PMR, Mass Spec
ORGANISM: *Aplysia dactylomela* (Mollusca)
REFERENCE: 421

$C_{15}H_{20}O$ Dehydrodendrolasin

MOL. WT.: 216
MELTING POINT: Oil
$[\alpha]_D$: 0
SPECTRAL DATA: UV, PMR, Mass Spec
ORGANISM: *Pleraplysilla spinifera* (Porifera)
REFERENCE: 99

$C_{15}H_{20}O$ Pallescensin-2

MOL. WT.: 216
MELTING POINT: Oil
$[\alpha]_D$: $+39.5$
SPECTRAL DATA: UV, IR, PMR, Mass Spec
ORGANISM: *Disidea pallescens* (Porifera)
REFERENCE: 87

$C_{15}H_{20}O$ Pallescensin B

MOL. WT.: 216
MELTING POINT: Oil
$[\alpha]_D$: $+62.6$
SPECTRAL DATA: UV, PMR, Mass Spec
ORGANISM: *Disidea pallescens* (Porifera)
REFERENCE: 85

C₁₅H₂₀O   Pleraplysillin

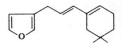

MOL. WT.: 216
MELTING POINT: Oil
[α]ᴅ: 0
SPECTRAL DATA: UV, PMR, Mass Spec
ORGANISM: *Pleraplysilla spinifera* (Porifera)
REFERENCE: 99

C₁₅H₂₀O₃   Pallescensin-3

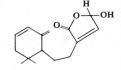

MOL. WT.: 248
MELTING POINT: Oil
SPECTRAL DATA: UV, IR, PMR
ORGANISM: *Disidea pallescens* (Porifera)
REFERENCE: 87

C₁₅H₂₁Br₂ClO₃   Prepacifenol

MOL. WT.: 445
MELTING POINT: 98–99°C; *p*-Bromobenzoate,
                297–298.5°C
SPECTRAL DATA: IR, PMR, Mass Spec
ORGANISM: *Aplysia californica* (Mollusca)
REFERENCE: 142

C₁₅H₂₂O   Dendrolasin

MOL. WT.: 218
MELTING POINT: Oil
SPECTRAL DATA: UV, IR, PMR, Mass Spec
ORGANISM: *Oligoceras hemorrhages* (Spongida)
REFERENCE: 422

C₁₅H₂₂O   Microcionin-1

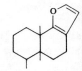

MOL. WT.: 218
MELTING POINT: Oil
[α]ᴅ: +7
SPECTRAL DATA: UV, PMR, Mass Spec
ORGANISM: *Microciona toxystila* (Porifera)
REFERENCE: 84

$C_{15}H_{22}O$ Microcionin-2

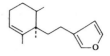

MOL. WT.:   218
MELTING POINT: Oil
$[\alpha]_D$:   −58.3
SPECTRAL DATA: UV, IR, PMR, Mass Spec
ORGANISM: *Microciona toxystila* (Porifera)
REFERENCE: 84

$C_{15}H_{22}O$ Microcionin-3

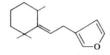

MOL. WT.:   218
MELTING POINT: Oil
$[\alpha]_D$:   +36.5
SPECTRAL DATA: UV, PMR, Mass Spec
ORGANISM: *Microciona toxystila* (Porifera)
REFERENCE: 84

$C_{15}H_{22}O$ Microcionin-4

MOL. WT.:   218
MELTING POINT: Oil
$[\alpha]_D$:   +98.3
SPECTRAL DATA: UV, IR, PMR, Mass Spec
ORGANISM: *Microciona toxystila* (Porifera)
REFERENCE: 84

$C_{15}H_{22}O$ Pallescensin-1

MOL. WT.:   218
MELTING POINT: Oil
SPECTRAL DATA: UV, IR, PMR, Mass Spec
ORGANISM: *Disidea pallescens* (Porifera)
REFERENCE: 87

$C_{15}H_{22}O$ Pallescensin A

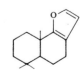

MOL.WT.:   218
MELTING POINT: Oil
SPECTRAL DATA: UV, PMR, Mass Spec
ORGANISM: *Disidea pallescens* (Porifera)
REFERENCE: 85

C₁₅H₂₄   9-Aristolene

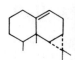

MOL. WT.:   204
[α]ᴅ: +80.9
SPECTRAL DATA: PMR, Mass Spec
ORGANISM: *Pseudopterogorgia americana* Gmelin
            (Coelenterata)
REFERENCE: 434

C₁₅H₂₄   1(10)-Aristolene

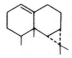

MOL. WT.:   204
[α]ᴅ: −78.5
SPECTRAL DATA: PMR, Mass Spec
ORGANISM: *Pseudopterogorgia americana* Gmelin
            (Coelenterata)
REFERENCE: 434

C₁₅H₂₄   (+)-β-Elemene

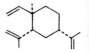

MOL. WT.:   204
[α]ᴅ: +15.1
SPECTRAL DATA: Mass Spec
ORGANISM: *Eunicea mammosa* Lamouroux
            (Coelenterata)
REFERENCE: 435

C₁₅H₂₄   (−)-Germacrene-A

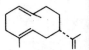

MOL. WT.:   204
[α]ᴅ: −3.2
SPECTRAL DATA: UV, IR, PMR, Mass Spec
ORGANISM: *Eunicea mammosa* Lamouroux
            (Coelenterata)
REFERENCE: 435

C$_{15}$H$_{24}$ β-Gorgonene

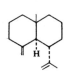

MOL. WT.:   204
MELTING POINT: AgNO$_3$ complex, 132.5–133.5°C
[α]$_D$:   +13.9
SPECTRAL DATA: IR, PMR, Mass Spec
ORGANISM: *Pseudopterogorgia americana* Gmelin
        (Coelenterata)
REFERENCE: 434

C$_{15}$H$_{24}$ (+)-γ-Maaliene

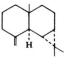

MOL. WT.:   204
MELTING POINT: Diol, 141–142°C
[α]$_D$:   +10.9   SOLVENT: He
SPECTRAL DATA: PMR, Mass Spec
ORGANISM: *Pseudopterogorgia americana* Gmelin
        (Coelenterata)
REFERENCE: 434

C$_{15}$H$_{24}$ (−)-β-Selinene

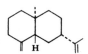

MOL. WT.:   204
ORGANISM: *Eunicea mammosa* Lamouroux
        (Coelenterata)
REFERENCE: 435

C$_{15}$H$_{24}$O$_2$ Dactyloxene B

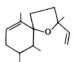

MOL. WT.:   236
MELTING POINT: Oil
[α]$_D$:   +106   SOLVENT: Chf
SPECTRAL DATA: UV, IR, PMR, Mass Spec
ORGANISM: *Aplysia dactylomela* (Mollusca)
REFERENCE: 366

$C_{15}H_{24}O_3$ $\Delta^{9(12)}$-Capnellene-3β,8β,10α-triol

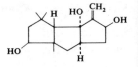

MOL. WT.: 252
MELTING POINT: 114–117°C; Diacetate, 91°C
$[\alpha]_D$: +2   SOLVENT: Chf
SPECTRAL DATA: IR, PMR, Mass Spec
ORGANISM: *Capnella imbricata* (Coelenterata)
REFERENCE: 210

$C_{15}H_{26}O$ Africanol

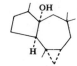

MOL. WT.: 222
MELTING POINT: 58–60°C
$[\alpha]_D$: +59.5   SOLVENT: Chf
SPECTRAL DATA: UV, IR, PMR, Mass Spec
ORGANISM: *Lemnalia africana* (Coelenterata)
REFERENCE: 412

$C_{16}H_{23}N$ Axisonitrile-4

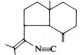

MOL. WT.: 229
MELTING POINT: 56–58°C
$[\alpha]_D$: 51.4   SOLVENT: Chf
SPECTRAL DATA: IR, PMR, Mass Spec
ORGANISM: *Axinella cannabina* (Porifera)
REFERENCE: 195

$C_{16}H_{23}NS$ Axisothiocyanate-4

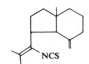

MOL. WT.: 261
$[\alpha]_D$: 35.9   SOLVENT: Chf
SPECTRAL DATA: IR, PMR, Mass Spec
ORGANISM: *Axinella cannabina* (Porifera)
REFERENCE: 195

$C_{16}H_{25}NO$ Axamide-4

MOL. WT.: 247
MELTING POINT: 81–84°C
$[\alpha]_D$: +63.3
SPECTRAL DATA: IR, PMR, Mass Spec
ORGANISM: *Axinella cannabina* (Porifera)
REFERENCE: 195

$C_{16}H_{26}O_2$ Methyl *trans*-monocyclofarnesate

MOL. WT.: 250
MELTING POINT: Oil (Acid 113–111°C)
SPECTRAL DATA: IR, PMR, Mass Spec
ORGANISM: *Halichondria panicea* (Porifera)
REFERENCE: 91

$C_{19}H_{40}$ Pristane

MOL. WT.: 268
MELTING POINT: Oil
REFERENCE: 25

$C_{20}H_{24}O_2$ Metanethole

MOL. WT.: 296
MELTING POINT: 135°C
ORGANISM: *Spheciospongia vesparia* (Porifera)
REFERENCE: 41

$C_{20}H_{24}O_4$ Pleraplysillin-2

MOL. WT.: 328
MELTING POINT: Oil
SPECTRAL DATA: UV, IR, PMR, Mass Spec
ORGANISM: *Pleraplysilla spinifera* (Porifera)
REFERENCE: 90

$C_{20}H_{28}O_3$ Lobophytolide

MOL. WT.: 316
MELTING POINT: 137–138°C
$[\alpha]_D$: +7   SOLVENT: Chf
SPECTRAL DATA: UV, IR, PMR, Mass Spec
ORGANISM: *Lobophytum cristagalli* von Marenzeller
            (Coelenterata)
REFERENCE: 413

C$_{20}$H$_{28}$O$_3$ **Sarcophine**

MOL. WT.:   316
MELTING POINT: 133–134°C
[α]$_D$:   +92   SOLVENT: Chf
SPECTRAL DATA: IR, PMR, Mass Spec
ORGANISM: *Sarcophytum glaucum* (Coelenterata)
REFERENCE: 46, 312

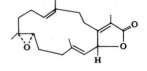

C$_{20}$H$_{28}$O$_3$

MOL. WT.:   316
MELTING POINT: 70°C
[α]$_D$:   −16   SOLVENT: MeOH
ORGANISM: *Sarcophytum glaucum* (Coelenterata)
REFERENCE: 215

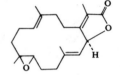

C$_{20}$H$_{28}$O$_3$

MOL. WT.:   316
MELTING POINT: Oil
SPECTRAL DATA: IR, PMR, Mass Spec
ORGANISM: *Sarcophytum glaucum* (Coelenterata)
REFERENCE: 215

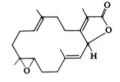

C$_{20}$H$_{30}$O$_2$ **Dictyol A**

MOL. WT.:   302
MELTING POINT: 84–86°C
[α]$_D$:   +79.6   SOLVENT: Chf
SPECTRAL DATA: PMR, Mass Spec
ORGANISM: *Aplysia depilans* (Mollusca)
REFERENCE: 295

C$_{20}$H$_{30}$O$_2$ **Dictyol B**

MOL. WT.:   302
MELTING POINT: 112–115°C
[α]$_D$:   +76   SOLVENT: Chf
SPECTRAL DATA: PMR, Mass Spec
ORGANISM: *Aplysia depilans* (Mollusca)
REFERENCE: 295

$C_{20}H_{30}O_2$ Isoagatholactone

MOL. WT.:   302
MELTING POINT: 153–155°C
$[\alpha]_D$:   +6.3
SPECTRAL DATA: UV, IR, PMR, Mass Spec
ORGANISM: *Spongia officinalis obliqua* (Porifera)
REFERENCE: 82

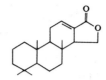

$C_{20}H_{30}O_2$

MOL. WT.:   302
MELTING POINT: Oil
$[\alpha]_D$:   +40   SOLVENT: Me
SPECTRAL DATA: IR, PMR, Mass Spec
ORGANISM: *Sarcophytum glaucum* (Coelenterata)
REFERENCE: 215

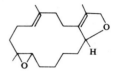

$C_{20}H_{30}O_2$

MOL. WT.:   302
MELTING POINT: Oil
SPECTRAL DATA: IR, Mass Spec
ORGANISM: *Sarcophytum glaucum* (Coelenterata)
REFERENCE: 215

$C_{20}H_{39}O_4$ Eunicin

MOL. WT.:   334
BIOACTIVITY: Antibacterial
MELTING POINT: 155°C; Iodoacetate, 149–150°C
$[\alpha]_D$:   −89
SPECTRAL DATA: IR
ORGANISM: *Eunicea mammosa* Lamouroux (Coelenterata)
REFERENCE: 189, 431

$C_{20}H_{30}O_4$ (15R)-15-Hydroxy-9-oxo-5-*cis*-10,13-*trans*-prostatrienoic acid

MOL. WT.:   334
ORGANISM: *Plexaura homomalla* (Coelenterata)
REFERENCE: 432

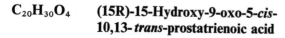

C$_{20}$H$_{30}$O$_4$ **(15S)-15-Hydroxy-9-oxo-*cis*-10,13-*trans*-prostatrienoic acid**

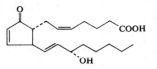

MOL. WT.: 334
ORGANISM: *Plexaura homomalla* (Coelenterata)
REFERENCE: 369

C$_{20}$H$_{30}$O$_4$ **(15S)-15-Hydroxy-9-oxo-5-*trans*-10,13-*trans*-prostatrienoic acid**

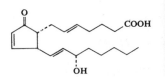

MOL. WT.: 334
MELTING POINT: Oil
[α]$_D$: +128   SOLVENT: Chf
SPECTRAL DATA: UV
ORGANISM: *Plexaura homomalla* (Coelenterata)
REFERENCE: 56

C$_{20}$H$_{30}$O$_4$ **Sinulariolide**

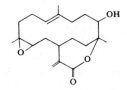

MOL. WT.: 334
MELTING POINT: 170–173°C
[α]$_D$: +76   SOLVENT: Me
SPECTRAL DATA: UV, IR, PMR, Mass Spec
ORGANISM: *Sinularia flexibilis* (Coelenterata)
REFERENCE: 414

C$_{20}$H$_{32}$ **Flexibilene**

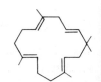

MOL. WT.: 272
MELTING POINT: Oil
[α]$_D$: 0
SPECTRAL DATA: UV, IR, PMR, Mass Spec
ORGANISM: *Sinularia flexibilis* (Coelenterata)
REFERENCE: 178

C$_{20}$H$_{32}$O   **6-Isopropyl-3,9,13-trimethylcyclo-tetradec-2,7,9,12-tetraene-1-ol**

MOL. WT.: 288
MELTING POINT: 143–145°C
SPECTRAL DATA: Mass Spec
ORGANISM: *Sarcophytum glaucum* (Coelenterata)
REFERENCE: 215

$C_{20}H_{32}O$ Pachydictyol A

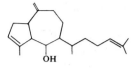

MOL. WT.: 288
MELTING POINT: Oil
$[\alpha]_D$: +104
SPECTRAL DATA: Mass Spec
ORGANISM: *Aplysia depilans* (Mollusca)
REFERENCE: 295

$C_{20}H_{32}O_3$ Asperdiol

MOL. WT.: 320
MELTING POINT: 109–110°C
$[\alpha]_D$: −87   SOLVENT: Chf
SPECTRAL DATA: IR, PMR, Mass Spec
ORGANISM: *Eunicea asperula, Eunicea tourneforti*
          (Coelenterata)
REFERENCE: 429

$C_{20}H_{34}O$ Nephthenol

MOL. WT.: 290
MELTING POINT: Oil
SPECTRAL DATA: IR, PMR, Mass Spec
ORGANISM: *Nephthea* sp. (Coelenterata)
REFERENCE: 368

$C_{20}H_{34}O_2$ 2-Hydroxynephthenol

MOL. WT.: 306
MELTING POINT: 98–99°C
$[\alpha]_D$: −104   SOLVENT: Chf
SPECTRAL DATA: UV, IR, PMR, Mass Spec
ORGANISM: *Litophyton viridis* (Coelenterata)
REFERENCE: 411

$C_{20}H_{34}O_2$ 6-Isopropyl-3,9,13-trimethylcyclo-tetradec-2,7,12-triene-1,9-diol

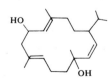

MOL. WT.: 306
MELTING POINT: Oil
SPECTRAL DATA: IR, PMR
ORGANISM: *Sarcophytum glaucum* (Coelenterata)
REFERENCE: 215

C$_{20}$H$_{35}$BrO$_2$ **Aplysin-20**

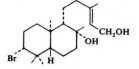

MOL. WT.:   387
MELTING POINT: 146–147°C; Acetate, 59–62°C
[α]$_D$: −78.1   SOLVENT: MeOH
SPECTRAL DATA: UV, IR, PMR, Mass Spec
ORGANISM: *Aplysia kurodai* (Mollusca)
REFERENCE: 289, 452

C$_{21}$H$_{24}$O$_4$ **Nitenin**

MOL. WT.: 340
MELTING POINT: Oil; Niteninic Acid, 89–95°C
[α]$_D$: −45.4   SOLVENT: Chf
SPECTRAL DATA: UV, IR, PMR, Mass Spec
ORGANISM: *Spongia nitens* (Porifera)
REFERENCE: 136

C$_{21}$H$_{24}$O$_6$ **Pukalide**

MOL. WT.: 372
MELTING POINT: 204–206°C
[α]$_D$: +44   SOLVENT: Chf
SPECTRAL DATA: UV, IR, PMR, Mass Spec
ORGANISM: *Sinularia abrupta* (Coelenterata)
REFERENCE: 301

C$_{21}$H$_{26}$O$_3$ **Furospongin-2**

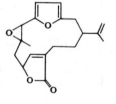

MOL. WT.: 326
MELTING POINT: Oil
[α]$_D$: 0
SPECTRAL DATA: UR, IR, PMR, Mass Spec
ORGANISM: *Spongia officinalis obliqua*, and
                   Hippospongia communis (Porifera)
REFERENCE: 96

C₂₁H₂₆O₃   Isofurospongin-2

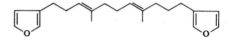

MOL. WT.: 326
MELTING POINT: Oil
SPECTRAL DATA: UV, IR, PMR, Mass Spec
ORGANISM: *Spongia officinalis obliqua*, and *Hippospongia communis*
    (Porifera)
REFERENCE: 96

C₂₁H₂₆O₄   Dihydronitenin

MOL. WT.: 342
MELTING POINT: Oil
[α]ᴅ: −25.2   SOLVENT: Chf
SPECTRAL DATA: UV, IR, PMR, Mass Spec
ORGANISM: *Spongia nitens* (Porifera)
REFERENCE: 136

C₂₁H₂₈O₂   Anhydrofurospongin-1

MOL. WT.: 312
MELTING POINT: Oil
[α]ᴅ: 0
SPECTRAL DATA: UV, IR, PMR, Mass Spec
ORGANISM: *Spongia officinalis obliqua*, and *Hippospongia communis*
    (Porifera)
REFERENCE: 96

C₂₁H₂₈O₂   Avarone

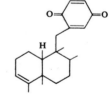

MOL. WT.: 312
MELTING POINT: Oil
SPECTRAL DATA: UV, IR
ORGANISM: *Disidea avora* (Porifera)
REFERENCE: 297

C₂₁H₂₈O₃   Dihydrofurospongin-2

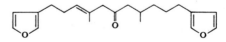

MOL. WT.: 328
MELTING POINT: Oil
[α]ᴅ: 0.91   SOLVENT: Chf
SPECTRAL DATA: UV, IR, PMR, Mass Spec
ORGANISM: *Spongia officinalis obliqua*, and *Hippospongia communis*
    (Porifera)
REFERENCE: 96

C$_{21}$H$_{28}$O$_4$ **Ircinin-3**

MOL. WT.:   344
MELTING POINT: Oil (isolated as methyl ester)
[α]$_D$:   +2.1   SOLVENT: Chf
SPECTRAL DATA: UV, IR, PMR, Mass Spec
ORGANISM: *Ircinia oros* (Porifera)
REFERENCE: 93

C$_{21}$H$_{28}$O$_4$ **Ircinin-4**

MOL. WT.:   344
MELTING POINT: Oil (isolated as methyl ester)
[α]$_D$:   −1.7   SOLVENT: Chf
SPECTRAL DATA: UV, IR, PMR, Mass Spec
ORGANISM: *Ircinia oros* (Porifera)
REFERENCE: 93

C$_{21}$H$_{30}$O$_2$ **Avarol**

MOL. WT.:   314
MELTING POINT: 148–150°C
[α]$_D$:   6.1   SOLVENT: Chf
SPECTRAL DATA: UV, IR, PMR, Mass Spec
ORGANISM: *Disidea avora* (Porifera)
REFERENCE: 111, 297

C$_{21}$H$_{30}$O$_2$ **ent-Chromazonarol**

MOL. WT.:   314
MELTING POINT: Gum; Acetate, 118–121°C
[α]$_D$:   +39   SOLVENT: Chf
SPECTRAL DATA: UV, IR, PMR, Mass Spec
ORGANISM: *Disidea pallescens* (Porifera)
REFERENCE: 88

$C_{21}H_{30}O_3$ Furospongin-1

MOL. WT.: 330
MELTING POINT: 35°C
$[\alpha]_D$: +8.8   SOLVENT: Chf
SPECTRAL DATA: UV, IR, PMR, Mass Spec
ORGANISM: *Spongia officinalis obliqua*, and *Hippospongia communis*
         (Porifera)
REFERENCE: 96, 97

$C_{21}H_{30}O_3$ Tetrahydrofurospongin-2

MOL. WT.: 330
MELTING POINT: Oil
$[\alpha]_D$: 0   SOLVENT: Chf
SPECTRAL DATA: UV, IR, PMR, Mass Spec
ORGANISM: *Spongia officinalis obliqua*, and *Hippospongia communis*
         (Porifera)
REFERENCE: 96

$C_{21}H_{34}O_5$ (15S)-11,15-Dihydroxy-9-oxo-5-*cis*-13-*trans*-prostadienoic acid

MOL. WT.: 366
ORGANISM: *Plexaura homomalla* (Coelenterata)
REFERENCE: 369

$C_{22}H_{30}O_5$ Lobolide

MOL. WT.: 374
MELTING POINT: 114–115°C
$[\alpha]_D$: −58   SOLVENT: Chf
SPECTRAL DATA: UV, IR, PMR, Mass Spec
ORGANISM: *Lobophytum* sp. (Coelenterata)
REFERENCE: 214

$C_{22}H_{32}O_5$ Crassin Acetate

MOL. WT.:   376
BIOACTIVITY: Antibiotic
MELTING POINT: 144–145.5°C
ORGANISM: *Pseudoplexaura porosa, Pseudoplexaura crassa,* and *Pseudoplexaura wagenaari* (Coelenterata)
REFERENCE: 190, 427

$C_{22}H_{34}O_4$ Ancepsenolide

MOL. WT.:   362
MELTING POINT: 91.5–92°C
SPECTRAL DATA: UV, IR, PMR, Mass Spec
ORGANISM: *Pterogorgia anceps* Pallas, and *Xiphigorgia anceps* (Coelenterata)
REFERENCE: 363

$C_{22}H_{36}O_3$ Epoxynephthenol Acetate

MOL. WT.:   348
MELTING POINT: Oil
$[\alpha]_D$:   −20.7
SPECTRAL DATA: UV, IR, PMR
ORGANISM: *Nephthea* sp. (Coelenterata)
REFERENCE: 368

$C_{22}H_{36}O_5$ Hydroxyancepsenolide

MOL. WT.:   380
MELTING POINT: 122.5–123.7°C; Acetate, 68.3–70.3°C
SPECTRAL DATA: UV, IR, PMR, Mass Spec
ORGANISM: *Pterogorgia anceps* Pallas (Coelenterata)
REFERENCE: 365

C$_{23}$H$_{24}$O$_5$　　Methyl (15R)-15-hydroxy-5-*cis*-10,13-*trans*-prostatrienoate 15-acetate

MOL. WT.: 380
SPECTRAL DATA: IR, PMR, Mass Spec
ORGANISM: *Plexaura homomalla* (Coelenterata)
REFERENCE: 432

C$_{24}$H$_{29}$O$_8$Cl　　Ptilosarcenone

MOL. WT.: 480
SPECTRAL DATA: UV, IR, PMR
ORGANISM: *Ptilosarcus gurneyi* (Gray)
　　　　　　(Coelenterata)
REFERENCE: 446

C$_{24}$H$_{44}$O$_5$　　Chondrillin

MOL. WT.: 412
MELTING POINT: 30°C
SPECTRAL DATA: PMR, Mass Spec
ORGANISM: *Chondrilla* sp. (Porifera)
REFERENCE: 437

C$_{25}$H$_{28}$O$_4$　　Icrinolide

MOL. WT.: 382
MELTING POINT: Oil
SPECTRAL DATA: UV, IR, PMR, Mass Spec
ORGANISM: *Thorecta marginalis* (Porifera)
REFERENCE: 223

$C_{25}H_{28}O_5$ **24-Hydroxyircinolide**

MOL. WT.: 408
MELTING POINT: Oil
SPECTRAL DATA: UV, IR, PMR, Mass Spec
ORGANISM: *Thorecta marginalis* (Porifera)
REFERENCE: 223

$C_{25}H_{30}O_5$ **Ircinin-1**

MOL. WT.: 410
MELTING POINT: Oil
SPECTRAL DATA: UV, IR, PMR, Mass Spec
ORGANISM: *Ircinia oros* (Porifera)
REFERENCE: 95

$C_{25}H_{30}O_5$ **Ircinin-2**

MOL. WT.: 410
SPECTRAL DATA: UV, IR, PMR, Mass Spec
ORGANISM: *Ircinia oros* (Porifera)
REFERENCE: 95

$C_{25}H_{34}O_4$ **Fasciculatin**

MOL. WT.: 398
MELTING POINT: Oil
$[\alpha]_D$: -15.60 SOLVENT: Chf
SPECTRAL DATA: UV, IR, PMR, Mass Spec
ORGANISM: *Ircinia fasciculata* (Porifera)
REFERENCE: 66

$C_{25}H_{34}O_4$ **Variabilin**

MOL. WT.: 398
MELTING POINT: Oil
SPECTRAL DATA: UV, IR, PMR
ORGANISM: *Ircinia variabilis* Schmidt (Porifera)
REFERENCE: 139

$C_{25}H_{58}O$ **Furospinosulin-1**

MOL. WT.: 354
MELTING POINT: Oil
SPECTRAL DATA: UV, PMR, Mass Spec
ORGANISM: *Ircinia spinosula* (Porifera)
REFERENCE: 94

$C_{26}H_{35}O_{10}Cl$ **Stylatulide**

MOL. WT.: 542
MELTING POINT: 179–181°C
$[\alpha]_D$: +65
SPECTRAL DATA: IR, PMR
ORGANISM: *Stylatula* sp. (Coelenterata)
REFERENCE: 445

$C_{26}H_{42}O_8$ **2-(13-Carboxy-14,15-diacetoxy-hexadecanyl)-2-penten-4-olide**

MOL. WT.: 482
BIOACTIVITY: Antibiotic
MELTING POINT: 81–82.9°C
$[\alpha]_D$: −8.3   SOLVENT: Chf
SPECTRAL DATA: UV, IR, PMR, Mass Spec
ORGANISM: *Pterogorgia quadalupensis* (Coelenterata)
REFERENCE: 364

$C_{27}H_{38}O_3$ **9-Hydroxy-3-tetrapyrenylbenzoic acid**

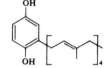

MOL. WT.:   410
MELTING POINT: 61–63°C
SPECTRAL DATA: UV, IR, PMR, Mass Spec
ORGANISM: *Ircinia muscarum* (Porifera)
REFERENCE: 92

$C_{27}H_{40}O_2$ **2-Tetraprenyl-1,4-benzoquinone**

MOL. WT.:   396
MELTING POINT: 47–48°C
SPECTRAL DATA: UV, IR, PMR, Mass Spec
ORGANISM: *Ircinia muscarum* (Porifera)
REFERENCE: 92

$C_{27}H_{40}O_4$ **Scalaradiol**

MOL. WT.:   428
MELTING POINT: 111–113°C
$[\alpha]_D$:   +47.3   SOLVENT: MeOH
SPECTRAL DATA: UV, IR, PMR, Mass Spec
ORGANISM: *Cacospongia mollior* (Porifera)
REFERENCE: 90

$C_{27}H_{40}O_5$ **Scalarin**

MOL. WT.:   444
MELTING POINT: 133–135°C
$[\alpha]_D$:   +43.2   SOLVENT: Chf
SPECTRAL DATA: UV, IR, PMR, Mass Spec
ORGANISM: *Cacospongia scalaris* (Porifera)
REFERENCE: 131

$C_{28}H_{37}O_{10}Cl$ **Ptilosarcone**

MOL. WT.:   568
MELTING POINT: Glass
SPECTRAL DATA: UV, IR, PMR
ORGANISM: *Ptilosarcus gurneyi* (Gray) (Coelenterata)
REFERENCE: 446

$C_{28}H_{42}O_9$ Eunicellin

MOL. WT.: 522
MELTING POINT: 186–188°; Dibromide, 211–213°C
$[\alpha]_D$: −36
SPECTRAL DATA: UV, IR, PMR, Mass Spec
ORGANISM: *Eunicella stricta* (Coelenterata)
REFERENCE: 228

$C_{30}H_{44}O_4$ 17-Desoxy-22,25-oxidoholothurinogenin

MOL. WT.: 468
MELTING POINT: 285.8–286.4°C; Acetate,
      266.2–266.5°C
$[\alpha]_D$: −9.3   SOLVENT: Chf
ORGANISM: *Actinopyga agassizi* and *Holothuria polii*
      (Echinodermata)
REFERENCE: 77, 169

$C_{30}H_{44}O_4$ Stichopogenin A_2

MOL. WT.: 468
MELTING POINT: 238–240°C; Monoacetate, 216–219°C
$[\alpha]_D$: −48   SOLVENT: Chf
SPECTRAL DATA: IR, PMR
ORGANISM: *Stichopus japonicus* Selenka
      (Echinodermata)
REFERENCE: 115, 408

$C_{30}H_{44}O_5$ 12α-Hydroxy-7,8-dihydro-24,25-dehydroholothurinogenin

MOL. WT.: 484
MELTING POINT: Diacetate, 240–243°C
ORGANISM: *Actinopyga agassizi* (Echinodermata)
REFERENCE: 78

$C_{30}H_{44}O_5$ 22,25-Oxido-holothurinogenin

MOL. WT.:   484

MELTING POINT: 315.2–315.8°C; Acetate, 289.2–
289.6°C; 3,5-Dinitrobenzoate,
300–301°C

$[\alpha]_D$:   −21.2   SOLVENT: Chf

SPECTRAL DATA: UV, IR

ORGANISM: *Actinopyga agassizi* and *Holothuria polii*
(Echinodermata)

REFERENCE: 77, 169

$C_{30}H_{46}O$ Furospinosulin-2

MOL. WT.:   422

MELTING POINT: Oil

SPECTRAL DATA: UV, PMR, Mass Spec

ORGANISM: *Ircinia spinosula* (Porifera)

REFERENCE: 94

$C_{30}H_{46}O_3$ Seychellogenin

MOL. WT.:   454

MELTING POINT: 234–238°C; Acetate, 211–213°C

$[\alpha]_D$:   −7

SPECTRAL DATA: UV, IR

ORGANISM: *Bohadschia koellikeri* (Echinodermata)

REFERENCE: 349

$C_{30}H_{46}O_4$ Holothurinogenin

MOL. WT.:   470

MELTING POINT: 277°C; 3-Acetate, 254–257°C

SPECTRAL DATA: UV, IR, PMR, Mass Spec

ORGANISM: *Holothuria polii* (Echinodermata)

REFERENCE: 169

$C_{30}H_{46}O_4$ Koellikerigenin

MOL. WT.: 470
MELTING POINT: 213–214°C; Monoacetate,
213–216°C
$[\alpha]_D$: −8
SPECTRAL DATA: UV, IR
ORGANISM: *Bohadschia koellikeri* (Echinodermata)
REFERENCE: 349

$C_{30}H_{46}O_5$ Griseogenin

MOL. WT.: 486
MELTING POINT: 285–287°C; Diacetate,
259–261°C
$[\alpha]_D$: −22   SOLVENT: Chf
SPECTRAL DATA: UV, IR, PMR, Mass Spec
ORGANISM: *Haloderima grisea* L. and *Holothuria polii*
(Echinodermata)
REFERENCE: 169, 416

$C_{30}H_{46}O_5$ Holotoxinogenin [Stichopogenin A_4, 3β,20ξ,25-trihydroxy-16-oxolanost-9(11)-ene-18-carboxylic acid lactone (18 → 20)]

MOL. WT.: 486
MELTING POINT: 238–241°C; Acetate, 221–223°C;
Diacetate, 212–216°C
$[\alpha]_D$: −97.6   SOLVENT: MeOH
SPECTRAL DATA: UV, IR, PMR, Mass Spec
ORGANISM: *Stichopus chloronotus* Brandt and *Stichopus
japonicus* Selenka (Echinodermata)
REFERENCE: 115, 238, 408

C$_{30}$H$_{50}$ *trans*-**Squalene**

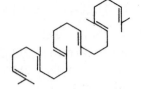

MOL. WT.: 410
ORGANISM: *Ircinia spinosula* (Porifera)
REFERENCE: 94

C$_{30}$H$_{52}$O   **Tetrahymanol**

MOL. WT.: 428
MELTING POINT: 312.5–314.5°C; Acetate, 303–305°C
SPECTRAL DATA: PMR
ORGANISM: *Tetrahymena pyriformis* (Protozoa)
REFERENCE: 284

C$_{31}$H$_{42}$O$_3$ **Paracentione**

MOL. WT.: 462
MELTING POINT: 147–149°C; Acetate
SPECTRAL DATA: UV, IR, PMR, Mass Spec
ORGANISM: *Paracentrotus lividus* Lam. (Echinodermata)
REFERENCE: 155

C$_{31}$H$_{44}$O$_2$ **Difurospinosulin**

MOL. WT.: 448
MELTING POINT: Oil
SPECTRAL DATA: UV, PMR, Mass Spec
ORGANISM: *Ircinia spinosula* (Porifera)
REFERENCE: 94

$C_{31}H_{48}O_4$ 25-Methoxy-17-desoxyholothurinogenin

MOL. WT.:   484
MELTING POINT: 242–245°C; 3-Acetate, 220°C
SPECTRAL DATA: UV, IR, PMR, Mass Spec
ORGANISM: *Holothuria polii* (Echinodermata)
REFERENCE: 169

$C_{31}H_{48}O_4$ Ternaygenin

MOL. WT.:   484
MELTING POINT: 239–242°C
$[\alpha]_D$:   +2
SPECTRAL DATA: UV, IR
ORGANISM: *Bohadschia koellikeri* (Echinodermata)
REFERENCE: 349

$C_{31}H_{48}O_5$ Holotoxinogenin 25-methyl ether

MOL. WT.:   500
MELTING POINT: 236–238°C; Acetate, 230–233°C
$[\alpha]_D$:   −125   SOLVENT: Me
SPECTRAL DATA: UV, IR, PMR, Mass Spec
ORGANISM: *Stichopus japonicus* Selenka
            (Echinodermata)
REFERENCE: 408

$C_{31}H_{48}O_5$ 12α-Methoxy-7,8-dihydro-17-desoxy-22,25-oxidoholothurinogenin

MOL. WT.:   500
MELTING POINT: Acetate, 205–208°C
ORGANISM: *Actinopyga agassizi* (Echinodermata)
REFERENCE: 78

$C_{31}H_{48}O_5$ **25-Methoxyholothurinogenin**
(Praslinogenin)

MOL. WT.:   500
MELTING POINT: 290–291.5°C; Monoacetate,
271–274°C
SPECTRAL DATA: UV, IR, PMR, Mass Spec
ORGANISM: *Holothuria polii* and *Bohadschia koellikeri*
(Echinodermata)
REFERENCE: 169, 415

$C_{31}H_{48}O_6$ **12β-Methoxy-7,8-dihydro-22,25-**
oxido-holothurinogenin

MOL. WT.:   516
MELTING POINT: Acetate, 273°C
ORGANISM: *Actinopyga agassizi* (Echinodermata)
REFERENCE: 78

$C_{31}H_{50}O_6$ **12β-Methoxy-7,8-dihydro-22-**
hydroxyholothurinogenin

MOL. WT.:   518
ORGANISM: *Actinopyga agassizi* (Echinodermata)
REFERENCE: 78

$C_{32}H_{50}O_5$ **23ξ-Acetoxy-17-deoxy-7,8-**
dihydroholothurinogenin

MOL. WT.:   514
MELTING POINT: 223–224°C; Me Acetate,
192–194°C
$[\alpha]_D$:   −20   SOLVENT: Chf
SPECTRAL DATA: IR, PMR, Mass Spec
ORGANISM: *Stichopus chloronotus* Brandt (Echinoder-
mata)
REFERENCE: 350

$C_{33}H_{50}O_6$ 17-Desoxy-12β-methoxy-7,8-dihydro-22,25-oxidoholothurinogenin-3-acetate

MOL. WT.: 542
MELTING POINT: 281–282°C
[α]$_D$: −45   SOLVENT: Chf
SPECTRAL DATA: UV, IR, PMR
ORGANISM: *Actinopyga agassizi* (Echinodermata)
REFERENCE: 79

$C_{33}H_{54}O_8$ 12β-Methoxy-7,8-dihydroholo-thurinogenin-3,22-diacetate

MOL. WT.: 578
MELTING POINT: 310°C
SPECTRAL DATA: UV, IR, PMR
ORGANISM: *Actinopyga agassizi* (Echinodermata)
REFERENCE: 79

$C_{34}H_{54}O_7$ 12β,25-Dimethoxy-7,8-dihydro-holothurinogenin-3-acetate

MOL. WT.: 574
MELTING POINT: 272–273°C
[α]$_D$: −51   SOLVENT: Chf
SPECTRAL DATA: UV, IR, PMR, Mass Spec
ORGANISM: *Actinopyga agassizi* (Echinodermata)
REFERENCE: 79

$C_{35}H_{54}O$ Furospinosulin-3

MOL. WT.: 490
MELTING POINT: Oil
SPECTRAL DATA: UV, IR, PMR, Mass Spec
ORGANISM: *Ircinia spinosula* (Porifera)
REFERENCE: 94

$C_{36}H_{54}O_2$ 2-Hexapyrenyl-1,4,quinol

MOL. WT.: 518
MELTING POINT: Oil
SPECTRAL DATA: UV, IR, PMR, Mass Spec
ORGANISM: *Ircinia spinosula* (Porifera)
REFERENCE: 94

$C_{36}H_{57}O_{10}$ 3β-Xyloside-12β-methoxy-7,8-
                            dihydro-24,25-dehydroholothurino-
                            genin

MOL. WT.: 649
SPECTRAL DATA: IR, PMR
ORGANISM: *Actinopyga agassizi*
            (Echinodermata)
REFERENCE: 78

$C_{37}H_{50}O_6$ 12β-Methoxy-7,8-dihydro-24,25-
                         dehydroholothurinogenin-3-acetate

MOL. WT.: 590
MELTING POINT: 245–247°C
$[\alpha]_D$: −53   SOLVENT: Chf
SPECTRAL DATA: IR, PMR
ORGANISM: *Actinopyga agassizi* (Echinodermata)
REFERENCE: 79

$C_{38}H_{48}O_2$ Alloxanthin (Cynthiaxanthin, pecten-
                         oxanthin)

MOL. WT.: 536
MELTING POINT: 188–190°C; Diacetate, 154–156°C
SPECTRAL DATA: UV, IR, PMR
ORGANISM: *Halocynthia papillosa* (Chordata/Tunicata)
REFERENCE: 67

$C_{38}H_{48}O_2$ Lutein (Xanthophyll)

MOL. WT.: 536
ORGANISM: *Chrysophrys major* Temminck
(Chordata/Pisces)
REFERENCE: 216, 217, 218

$C_{38}H_{52}O_2$ Zeaxanthin

MOL. WT.: 540
ORGANISM: *Chrysophrys major* Temminck
(Chordata/Pisces)
REFERENCE: 216

$C_{39}H_{50}O_7$ Peridinin

MOL. WT.: 630
MELTING POINT: 107–109°C
SPECTRAL DATA: UV, PMR, Mass Spec
ORGANISM: *Anthopleura xanthogrammica* (Coelenterata), *Cachonina niei*
(Pyrrophyta), and *Amphidinium operculatum* (Protozoa)
REFERENCE: 401

$C_{40}H_{48}$ Isorenieratene

MOL. WT.: 528
MELTING POINT: 199°C
SPECTRAL DATA: UV, IR
ORGANISM: *Reniera japonica* (Porifera)
REFERENCE: 447, 449, 451

$C_{40}H_{48}$ Renieratene

MOL. WT.:   528
MELTING POINT: 185°C
SPECTRAL DATA: UV, IR
ORGANISM: *Reniera japonica* (Porifera)
REFERENCE: 448, 449, 450, 451

$C_{40}H_{48}O_4$ Astacin

MOL. WT.:   592
ORGANISM: *Chrysophrys major* Temminck
                (Chordata/Pisces)
REFERENCE: 216

$C_{40}H_{48}O_4$ 7,7′8,8′-Tetradehydroastaxanthin

MOL. WT.:   592
MELTING POINT: 210°C
SPECTRAL DATA: UV, PMR, Mass Spec
ORGANISM: *Asterias rubens* (Echinodermata)
REFERENCE: 148

$C_{40}H_{50}O_4$ 7,8-Didehydroastaxanthin
(Asterinsäure)

MOL. WT.:   594
ORGANISM: *Asterias rubens* (Echinodermata)
REFERENCE: 148

$C_{40}H_{52}O_2$ **Cantharanthin (β-Carotene-4,4′-dione)**

MOL. WT.: 564
SPECTRAL DATA: UV
ORGANISM: *Stichopus japonicus* Selenka
(Echinodermata)
REFERENCE: 290

$C_{40}H_{52}O_3$ **α-Doradecin**

MOL. WT.: 580
ORGANISM: *Chrysophrys major* Temminck and
Crassius auratus (Chordata/Pisces)
REFERENCE: 216, 217, 218

$C_{40}H_{52}O_3$ **Pectenolone**

MOL. WT.: 580
ORGANISM: *Pecten maximus* (Mollusca) and
Halocynthia papillosa (Chordata/Tunicata)
REFERENCE: 67

$C_{40}H_{52}O_4$ **Astaxanthin**

MOL. WT.: 596
MELTING POINT: Diacetate 198–199°C
REFERENCE: 67

$C_{40}H_{54}O$ Echinenone

MOL. WT.: 550
MELTING POINT: 192–193°C
SPECTRAL DATA: UV
ORGANISM: *Chrysophrys major* Temminck
(Chordata/Pisces) and *Hymeniacidon
sanguineum* Grant (Porifera)
REFERENCE: 114, 216

$C_{40}H_{56}$ α-Carotene

MOL. WT.: 536
MELTING POINT: 185°C
SPECTRAL DATA: UV
ORGANISM: *Chrysophrys major* Temminck
(Chordata/Pisces) and *Reniera japonica*
(Porifera)
REFERENCE: 114, 216, 451

$C_{40}H_{56}$ β-Carotene

MOL. WT.: 536
MELTING POINT: 183°C
SPECTRAL DATA: UV
ORGANISM: *Chrysophrys major* Temminck
(Chordata/Pisces), *Reniera japonica*, and
Hymeniacidon sanguineum Grant (Porifera)
REFERENCE: 114, 216, 451

$C_{40}H_{56}$ γ-Carotene

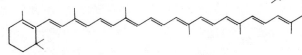

MOL. WT.: 536
MELTING POINT: 176–177°C
SPECTRAL DATA: UV
ORGANISM: *Hymeniacidon sanguineum* Grant (Porifera)
REFERENCE: 114

$C_{40}H_{56}O_2$ **3,3'-Dihydroxy-ε-carotene**

MOL. WT.: 568
ORGANISM: *Chrysophrys major* Temminck
(Chordata/Pisces)
REFERENCE: 216

$C_{40}H_{56}O_5$ **Fucoxanthinol**

MOL. WT.: 616
MELTING POINT: 134–138°C
SPECTRAL DATA: UV, IR, PMR, Mass Spec
ORGANISM: *Paracentrotus lividus* Lam.
(Echinodermata)
REFERENCE: 155

$C_{40}H_{60}O_2$ **Provitamine A (Kitol)**

MOL. WT.: 572
MELTING POINT: 135–136°C; Diacetate, 150–151°C
$[\alpha]_D$: −2.6 SOLVENT: Chf
SPECTRAL DATA: IR, PMR
REFERENCE: 160

$C_{65}H_{106}O_{27}$ **Holotoxin A**

MOL. WT.: 1318
MELTING POINT: 248–250°C
SPECTRAL DATA: UV, IR
ORGANISM: *Stichopus japonicus* Selenka
             (Echinodermata)
REFERENCE: 237

Chapter 12

Carbohydrates

C$_5$H$_{10}$O$_5$ **D-Xylose**

MOL. WT.: 150
MELTING POINT: 148–151°C
ORGANISM: *Stichopus japonicus, Holothuria tabulosa,*
and *Actinopyga agassizi* (Echinodermata)
REFERENCE: 22, 76, 79, 116, 170

C$_6$H$_{12}$O$_5$ **D-Quinovose (6-Deoxy-D-Glucose,**
D-Glucomethylose, Glumethylose)

MOL. WT.: 164
MELTING POINT: 146°C
ORGANISM: *Holothuria tabulosa* and *Actinopyga*
agassizi (Echinodermata)
REFERENCE: 22, 76, 79, 170

C$_6$H$_{12}$O$_6$ **D–Galactose**

MOL. WT.: 180
MELTING POINT: 165–168°C
ORGANISM: *Stichopus japonicus* Selenka
(Echinodermata)
REFERENCE: 116

$C_6H_{12}O_6$ D-Glucose

MOL. WT.:   180
MELTING POINT: 146°C
ORGANISM: *Actinopyga agassizi, Stichopus japonicus*
            Selenka, and *Holothuria tabulosa*
            (Echinodermata)
REFERENCE: 22, 76, 79, 116, 170

$C_6H_{12}O_6$ Inositol

MOL. WT.:   180
MELTING POINT: 247–248°C
$[\alpha]_D$:   +65
ORGANISM: *Calyx nicacensis* and *Geodia gigas*
            (Porifera)
REFERENCE: 10, 16

$C_7H_{14}O_6$ 3-Methoxy-D-Glucose (3-*O*-Methyl-glucose)

MOL. WT.:   194
ORGANISM: *Actinopyga agassizi, Stichopus japonicus*
            Selenka, and *Holothuria tabulosa*
            (Echinodermata)
REFERENCE: 22, 76, 79, 116, 170

Chapter 13

Phenols, Quinones, and Related Compounds

$C_6H_3Br_3O$ 2,4,6-Tribromophenol

MOL. WT.: 331
MELTING POINT: 95°C
SPECTRAL DATA: UV, PMR, Mass Spec
ORGANISM: *Phoronopsis viridis* Hilton (Phoronidea)
REFERENCE: 380

$C_6H_4Br_2O$ 2,6-Dibromophenol

MOL. WT.: 252
MELTING POINT: 51–52°C
SPECTRAL DATA: UV, PMR, Mass Spec
ORGANISM: *Balanoglossus biminiensis* (Chordata/
Hemichordata) and *Phoronopsis viridis*
Hilton (Phoronidea)
REFERENCE: 24, 380

$C_7H_4Br_2O_2$ 3,5-Dibromo-4-hydroxybenzaldehyde

MOL. WT.: 280
MELTING POINT: 182–186°C
ORGANISM: *Thelepus setosus* (Annelida)
REFERENCE: 179, 180

$C_7H_6Br_2O_2$ 3,5-Dibromo-4-hydroxybenzyl alcohol

MOL. WT.: 282
MELTING POINT: 115–116°C
ORGANISM: *Thelepus setosus* (Annelida)
REFERENCE: 179, 180

$C_8H_7Br_2NO_3$ 3-Acetamido-2,6-dibromo-3-hydroxy-2,6-cyclohexadiene-1-one

MOL. WT.: 325
BIOACTIVITY: Antibiotic
MELTING POINT: 193–195°C (dec.); Acetate, 185°C
SPECTRAL DATA: UV, IR, PMR, Mass Spec
ORGANISM: *Verongia fistularis* and *Verongia cauliformis*
          (Porifera)
REFERENCE: 374, 375

$C_8H_7Br_2NO_3$ 2,6-Dibromo-3-acetamidohydroquinone

MOL. WT.: 325
MELTING POINT: 170–172°C
SPECTRAL DATA: UV, IR, Mass Spec
ORGANISM: *Verongia aurea* Hyatt (Porifera)
REFERENCE: 252

$C_8H_8O_4$ 2,5-Dihydroxy-3-ethylbenzoquinone

MOL. WT.: 168
MELTING POINT: 130–145°C
SPECTRAL DATA: UV, IR, PMR, Mass Spec
ORGANISM: *Echinothrix diadema* Linn. (Echinodermata)
REFERENCE: 308

$C_{10}H_6O_5$ Naphthopurpurin

MOL. WT.: 206
MELTING POINT: 200–210°C
SPECTRAL DATA: UV
ORGANISM: *Echinothrix diadema* Linn. and
          Echinothrix calamaris Pallis
          (Echinodermata)
REFERENCE: 308, 390

$C_{10}H_6O_6$ 2,7-Dihydroxynaphthazarin

MOL. WT.: 222
MELTING POINT: 265–275°C; 2,7-Dimethoxy, 273-275°C
ORGANISM: *Echinothrix diadema* Linn. and *Echinothrix calamaris* Pallis (Echinodermata)
REFERENCE: 308

$C_{10}H_6O_6$ Spinochrome B

MOL. WT.: 222
MELTING POINT: 325–330°C; 2,3-Dimethoxy-7-hydroxy-juglone, 204–205°C; Leucoacetate, 242°C; Trimethyl Ether, 112°C; Tetramethyl Ether, 130–130.5°C; Tetra-acetate, 157°C
SPECTRAL DATA: UV
ORGANISM: *Echinothrix diadema* Linn., *Echinothrix calamaris* Pallis, *Salmacis sphaeroides*, *Paracentrotus lividus* Lam., *Echinus esculentus*, *Strongylocentrotus sulcherrimus*, and *Anthocidaris cassispina* (Echinodermata)
REFERENCE: 164, 308, 390

$C_{10}H_6O_7$ Spinochrome D

MOL. WT.: 238
MELTING POINT: 285–290°C; Penta-acetate, 179–180°C; 2,3,6-Trimethoxynaphthazarin, 161–162°C
SPECTRAL DATA: UV, IR
ORGANISM: *Echinothrix diadema* Linn. and *Echinothrix calamaris* Pallis (Echinodermata)
REFERENCE: 21, 308, 390

$C_{10}H_6O_8$ Spinochrome E

MOL. WT.: 254
MELTING POINT: 320°C; Hexa-acetate, 192°C; Leucoocta-acetate, 265°C
SPECTRAL DATA: UV
ORGANISM: *Psammechinus miliaris* Gmelin (Echinodermata)
REFERENCE: 396

$C_{10}H_{13}Br_2NO_4$ 3-Acetamido-2,6-dibromo-3-
hydroxy-1,1-dimethoxycyclohexa-
2,6-diene

MOL. WT.: 371
MELTING POINT: 191°C; Acetate, 184°C
SPECTRAL DATA: IR, PMR, Mass Spec
ORGANISM: *Verongia fistularis* and *Verongia
cauliformis* (Porifera)
REFERENCE: 374, 377

$C_{11}H_8O_8$ Namakochrome

MOL. WT.: 268
MELTING POINT: 218°C; Penta-acetyl, 158–163°C
SPECTRAL DATA: UV, IR
ORGANISM: *Polycheira rufescens* (Echinodermata)
REFERENCE: 310, 311

$C_{11}H_{15}Br_2NO_4$

MOL. WT.: 385
SPECTRAL DATA: Mass Spec
ORGANISM: *Verongia* sp. (Porifera)
REFERENCE: 20

$C_{12}H_5Br_5O_2$ 1,2,3,1′,3′-Pentabromo-5-
hydroxphenyl ether

MOL. WT.: 581
MELTING POINT: 185–186°C
SPECTRAL DATA: UV, IR, PMR, Mass Spec
ORGANISM: *Disidea herbacea* (Porifera)
REFERENCE: 376

$C_{12}H_8O_6$ 2,7-Dihydroxy-6-acetyljuglone

MOL. WT.: 248
MELTING POINT: 215°C (dec.)
SPECTRAL DATA: Mass Spec
ORGANISM: *Echinothrix diadema* Linn. and
Echinothrix calamaris Pallis
(Echinodermata)
REFERENCE: 31, 308

C₁₂H₈O₆ 2-Hydroxy-3-acetylnaphthazarin

MOL. WT.: 248
MELTING POINT: 163–164°C (dec.)
ORGANISM: *Echinothrix diadema* Linn. and
Echinothrix calamaris Pallis
(Echinodermata)
REFERENCE: 31, 308

C₁₂H₈O₇ Spinochrome A

MOL. WT.: 264
MELTING POINT: 192–193°C
SPECTRAL DATA: UV, PMR, Mass Spec
ORGANISM: *Echinothrix diadema* Linn., *Echinothrix
calamaris* Pallis, and *Paracentrotus
lividus* Lam. (Echinodermata)
REFERENCE: 31, 74, 75, 308

C₁₂H₈O₇ Spinochrome G

MOL. WT. 264
MELTING POINT: > 360°C
SPECTRAL DATA: UV, PMR, Mass Spec
REFERENCE: 162

C₁₂H₈O₇ Spinochrome S

MOL. WT.: 264
MELTING POINT: 275–280°C (dec.)
SPECTRAL DATA: UV, IR, PMR, Mass Spec
ORGANISM: *Salmacis sphaeroides* (Echinodermata)
REFERENCE: 163

C₁₂H₈O₇ 2,3,7-Trihydroxy-6-acetyljuglone

MOL. WT.: 264
MELTING POINT: 245–255°C; 2,3-Dimethoxy-7-
hydroxy-6-acetyljuglone, 134–135°C
SPECTRAL DATA: UV, Mass Spec
ORGANISM: *Echinothrix diadema* Linn. and *Echinothrix
calmaris* Pallis (Echinodermata)
REFERENCE: 162, 308

$C_{12}H_8Br_2O_2$ **4′,6-Dibromo-2-hydroxydiphenyl ether**

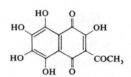

MOL. WT.:   344
MELTING POINT: 95–98°C
SPECTRAL DATA: UV, IR, PMR, Mass Spec
ORGANISM: *Disidea herbacea* (Porifera)
REFERENCE: 376

$C_{12}H_8O_8$ **Spinochrome C**

MOL. WT.:   280
MELTING POINT: 246–248°C; Trimethylether,
                         116–117°C
SPECIAL DATA: UV, IR, PMR
ORGANISM: *Echinometra oblonga, Echinothrix diadema*
                 Linn., and *Echinothrix calamaris*
                 (Echinodermata)
REFERENCE: 75, 308

$C_{12}H_{10}O_4$ **2-Hydroxy-6-ethyljuglone**

MOL. WT.:   218
MELTING POINT: 219–220°C
ORGANISM: *Echinothrix calamaris* Pallis
                 (Echinodermata)
REFERENCE: 308

$C_{12}H_{10}O_5$ **2-Hydroxy-3-ethylnaphthazarin**

MOL. WT.:   234
MELTING POINT: 185–186°C
ORGANISM: *Ophiocoma erinaceus* and *Ophiocoma*
                 insularia (Echinodermata)
REFERENCE: 389

$C_{12}H_{10}O_5$ **2-Hydroxy-6-ethylnaphthazarin**

MOL. WT.:   234
MELTING POINT: 204–204.5°C
ORGANISM: *Echinothrix calamaris* Pallis
                 (Echinodermata)
REFERENCE: 308

$C_{12}H_{10}O_6$ 2,7-Dihydroxy-3-ethylnaphthazarin

MOL. WT.: 250
MELTING POINT: 190–192°C; 2,7-Dimethoxy, 145–
147°C; 7-Methoxy, 230–232°C
ORGANISM: *Echinothrix diadema* Linn. and *Echinothrix
calamaris* Pallis (Echinodermata)
REFERENCE: 308

$C_{12}H_{10}O_6$ 2,3,7-Trihydroxy-6-ethyljuglone

MOL. WT.: 250
MELTING POINT: 265–269°C (dec.); Trimethylether,
113–114°C
SPECTRAL DATA: UV, PMR, Mass Spec
ORGANISM: *Echinothrix diadema* Linn. and *Echinothrix
calamaris* Pallis (Echinodermata)
REFERENCE: 308

$C_{12}H_{10}O_6$ 2,6,7-Trihydroxy-3-ethyljuglone

MOL. WT.: 250
MELTING POINT: 220–226°C
ORGANISM: *Ophiocoma erinaceus* and *Ophiocoma
insularia* (Echinodermata)
REFERENCE: 389

$C_{12}H_{10}O_8$ 2,6-Dihydroxy-3,7-dimethoxynaph-
thazarin

MOL. WT.: 282
MELTING POINT: 252–254°C
ORGANISM: *Acanthaster planci* Linn. (Echinodermata)
REFERENCE: 389

$C_{12}H_{10}O_8$ 2,7-Dihydroxy-3,6-dimethoxy-
naphthazarin

MOL. WT.: 282
MELTING POINT: 218–219°C
ORGANISM: *Acanthaster planci* Linn. (Echinodermata)
REFERENCE: 389

$C_{12}H_{12}O_7$ **Echinochrome A**

MOL. WT.: 268

MELTING POINT: 222–223°C; 2,3,6-Trimethoxy,
131–132°C; 3,7-Dimethoxy, 152–
154°C

SPECTRAL DATA: UV

ORGANISM: *Echinothrix diadema* Linn. and
Echinothrix calamaris Pallis (Echinodermata)

REFERENCE: 254, 308

$C_{13}H_8Br_4O_2$ **Bis-(3,5-dibromo-4-hydroxyphenyl)-
methane**

MOL. WT.: 516

MELTING POINT: 230–232°C

SPECTRAL DATA: UV, IR, PMR, Mass Spec

ORGANISM: *Thelepus setosus* (Annelida)

REFERENCE: 179

$C_{13}H_{10}O_7$ **2-Hydroxy-3-acetyl-7-methoxy-
naphthazarin**

MOL. WT.: 278

MELTING POINT: 246–248°C

ORGANISM: *Ophiocoma erinaceus* and *Ophiocoma
insularia* (Echinodermata)

REFERENCE: 389

$C_{13}H_{12}O_7$ **6-Ethyl-2,7-dihydroxy-2-methoxy-
naphthazarin**

MOL. WT.: 280

MELTING POINT: 202–204°C

SPECTRAL DATA: UV, IR, PMR, Mass Spec

ORGANISM: *Diadema antillarum* (Echinodermata)

REFERENCE: 288

$C_{14}H_{10}O_6$ 2-Methyl-8-hydroxy-2H-pyrano(3,2-g)-naphthazarin

MOL. WT.: 274
MELTING POINT: 165–172°C (dec.)
SPECTRAL DATA: UV, PMR, Mass Spec
ORGANISM: *Echinothrix diadema* Linn. and
Echinothrix calamaris Pallis (Echinodermata)
REFERENCE: 307

$C_{14}H_{11}Br_3O_3$

MOL. WT.: 467
MELTING POINT: 180–182°C
ORGANISM: *Thelepus setosus* (Annelida)
REFERENCE: 180

$C_{15}H_{12}O_5$ Anhydrofonsecin

MOL. WT.: 272
MELTING POINT: 268°C
SPECTRAL DATA: UV, IR, PMR, Mass Spec
ORGANISM: *Comantheria perplexa* (Echinodermata)
REFERENCE: 229

$C_{16}H_{12}O_4$ Hallachrome

MOL. WT.: 268
MELTING POINT: 224–226°C (dec.); Leucotriacetate,
148–149°C; Acetate, 194–196°C
SPECTRAL DATA: UV, PMR, Mass Spec
ORGANISM: *Halla parthenopeia* (Annelida)
REFERENCE: 345

C₁₆H₁₃NaO₈S   **Sodium comantheryl sulfate**

MOL. WT.: 388
SPECTRAL DATA: UV, IR, PMR
ORGANISM: *Comantheria perplexa* (Echinodermata)
REFERENCE: 229

C₁₆H₁₄O₅   **Comantherin**

MOL. WT.: 286
MELTING POINT: 272°C; Acetate, 220°C; Methyl ether,
                187–189°C and 178–179°C
SPECTRAL DATA: UV, IR, PMR, Mass Spec
ORGANISM: *Comantheria perplexa* (Echinodermata)
REFERENCE: 229

C₁₇H₁₂O₆   **3-Propionyl-1,6,8-trihydroxy-9,10-**
                anthraquinone

MOL. WT.: 312
MELTING POINT: 265–266°C
SPECTRAL DATA: UV, IR, PMR, Mass Spec
ORGANISM: *Comanthus bennetti* (Echinodermata)
REFERENCE: 30, 343

C₁₇H₁₄O₅   **3-Propyl-1,6,8-trihydroxy-9,10-**
                anthraquinone

MOL. WT.: 298
MELTING POINT: 219–221°C
SPECTRAL DATA: UV, IR, PMR, Mass Spec
ORGANISM: *Comanthus bennetti* (Echinodermata)
REFERENCE: 30

$C_{17}H_{14}O_6$

MOL. WT.: 314
SPECTRAL DATA: UV, IR, Mass Spec
ORGANISM: *Comanthus bennetti* (Echinodermata)
REFERENCE: 30

$C_{17}H_{14}O_6$ **Isochodoptilometrin**

MOL. WT.: 314
MELTING POINT: 275–277°C; 6-Methyl ether, 196–197°C;
Tetra-acetate, 161–162°C; Dimethyl ether, 136–137°C;
Trimethyl ether, 162–163°C
SPECTRAL DATA: UV, IR
ORGANISM: *Ptilometra australis* Wilton
(Echinodermata)
REFERENCE: 343

$C_{17}H_{14}O_6$ **S(—)-1,6,8-Trihydroxy-3-(1-hydroxypropyl)-anthraquinone (Rhodoptilometrin)**

MOL. WT.: 314
MELTING POINT: 217–218°C; Tetra-acetate, 156–157°C;
6-Methyl ether, 197–198°C; Tetramethyl
ether, 195–195.5°C; Leucotriacetyl
trimethyl ether, 204–206°C
SPECTRAL DATA: UV, IR, PMR, Mass Spec
ORGANISM: *Ptilometra australis* Wilton and *Comanthus
bennetti* (Echinodermata)
REFERENCE: 30, 343

$C_{17}H_{16}O_5$ Comaparvin

MOL. WT.: 300
MELTING POINT: 232–233°C (dec.); Acetate, 185–186°C;
                Dimethyl ether, 142–143°C
SPECTRAL DATA: UV, IR, Mass Spec
ORGANISM: *Comanthus parvicirrus timorensis* J. Müller
           (Echinodermata)
REFERENCE: 395

$C_{17}H_{16}O_{11}S_2$ Comaparvin-3,6-disulfate ester

(or monosulfate)

MOL. WT.: 460
ORGANISM: *Comanthus parvicirrus timorensis* J. Müller
           (Echinodermata)
REFERENCE: 395

$C_{18}H_{14}O_7$ Ptilometric acid

MOL. WT.: 342
MELTING POINT: 298–299°C; Triacetate, 194–195°C;
                Trimethyl ether; Methyl ester, 155–
                156°C
SPECTRAL DATA: UV, IR
ORGANISM: *Ptilometra australis* Wilton and *Tropiometra*
           afra Hartlaub (Echinodermata)
REFERENCE: 343

$C_{18}H_{18}O_5$ Neocemantherin

MOL. WT.: 314
MELTING POINT: 237°C (dec.); Acetate, 178–179°C;
                Methyl ether, 155–157°C
SPECTRAL DATA: IR, PMR, Mass Spec
ORGANISM: *Comantheria perplexa* (Echinodermata)
REFERENCE: 229

$C_{18}H_{18}O_6$ **5-Methoxy-comaparvin**

MOL. WT.: 330

MELTING POINT: 200–201.5°C; Dimethyl ether, 93–94°C; Methyl ether, 120–121°C; Monoacetate, 190–191°C; Diacetate, 171–173°C

SPECTRAL DATA: UV, IR, Mass Spec

ORGANISM: *Comanthus parvicirrus timorensis* J. Müller (Echinodermata)

REFERENCE: 395

$C_{18}H_{18}O_{12}S_2$ **5-Methoxy-comaparvin 3,6-disulfate ester**

MOL. WT.: 490

ORGANISM: *Comanthus parvicirrus timorensis* J. Müller (Echinodermata)

REFERENCE: 395

$C_{19}H_{16}O_7$ **Rhodocomatulin 6-monomethyl ether**

MOL. WT.: 356

MELTING POINT: 250–252°C (dec.); Triacetate, 194–196°C

SPECTRAL DATA: UV, IR

ORGANISM: *Comatula pectinata* Linn. and *Comatula cratera* Clark (Echinodermata)

REFERENCE: 404

$C_{19}H_{16}O_8$ **Rubrocomatulin monomethyl ether**

MOL. WT.: 372

MELTING POINT: 298–299°C (dec.); Tetra-acetate, 203–205°C; Pentamethyl ether, 152–153.5 and 214–215°C

ORGANISM: *Comatula pectinata* Linn. and *Comatula cratera* Clark (Echinodermata)

REFERENCE: 344

$C_{19}H_{18}O_6$

MOL. WT.: 342
SPECTRAL DATA: UV, IR, PMR, Mass Spec
ORGANISM: *Comanthus bennetti* (Echinodermata)
REFERENCE: 30

$C_{19}H_{20}O_6$ **5-Methoxycomaparvin 6-Methyl ether**

MOL. WT.: 344
MELTING POINT: 221–222°C; Methyl ether, 93–94°C;
Acetate, 129–130°C
SPECTRAL DATA: UV, IR, Mass Spec
ORGANISM: *Comanthus parvicirrus timorensis* J. Müller
(Echinodermata)
REFERENCE: 395

$C_{19}H_{20}O_9S$ **5-Methoxycomaparvin 6-Methyl ether 3-sulfate ester**

MOL. WT. 424
ORGANISM: *Comanthus parvicirrus timorensis*
J. Müller (Echinodermata)
REFERENCE: 395

$C_{20}H_{18}O_7$ **Rhodocomatulin 6,8-dimethyl ether**

MOL. WT.: 370
MELTING POINT: 229.5–230.5°C; Diacetate, 199.5–
201°C; Monobromide 222.5–223.5°C;
Dimethanesulfonyl ester, 248–250°C;
Oxime, 225°C
SPECTRAL DATA: UV, IR
ORGANISM: *Comatula pectinata* Linn. and *Comatula cratera* Clark (Echinodermata)
REFERENCE: 404

$C_{21}H_{12}O_6$ Arenicochrome

MOL. WT.: 360
MELTING POINT: Triacetate, 210–211°C
SPECTRAL DATA: IR
ORGANISM: *Arenicola marina* (Annelida)
REFERENCE: 309

$C_{22}H_{12}O_{13}$ Anhydroethylidene-3,3′-bis-(2,6,7-trihydroxynaphthazarin)

MOL. WT.: 484
MELTING POINT: 253–256°C
SPECTRAL DATA: UV, IR, Mass Spec
ORGANISM: *Spatangus purpurens* (Echinodermata)
REFERENCE: 288

$C_{22}H_{14}O_{14}$ Ethylidene-3,3′-bis(2,6,7-trihydroxy-naphthazarin)

MOL. WT.: 502
MELTING POINT: 155–157°C
SPECTRAL DATA: UV, IR, PMR
ORGANISM: *Spatangus purpurens* (Echinodermata)
REFERENCE: 288

$C_{32}H_{47}BrO_{10}$ Aplysiatoxin

MOL. WT.: 671
BIOACTIVITY: LD_{100} 0.3 mg/kg (mouse)
MELTING POINT: Oil
SPECTRAL DATA: UV, PMR, Mass Spec
ORGANISM: *Stylocheilus longicauda* (Quoy and Gaimard) (Mollusca)
REFERENCE: 219, 220

$C_{32}H_{48}O_{10}$ **Debromoaplysiatoxin**

MOL. WT.: 592
MELTING POINT: Oil
SPECTRAL DATA: PMR, Mass Spec
ORGANISM: *Stylocheilus longicauda* (Quoy
and Gaimard) (Mollusca)
REFERENCE: 219, 220

$C_{34}H_{49}BrO_{11}$

MOL. WT.: 713
ORGANISM: *Stylocheilus longicauda* (Quoy
and Gaimard (Mollusca)
REFERENCE: 219, 220

$C_{34}H_{50}O_{11}$

MOL. WT.: 634
ORGANISM: *Stylocheilus longicauda* (Quoy and
Gaimard) (Mollusca)
REFERENCE: 219, 220

$C_{36}H_{52}O_2$ **2-Hexapyrenyl-1,4-benzoquinone**

MOL. WT.: 516
MELTING POINT: Oil
SPECTRAL DATA: UV, IR, PMR, Mass Spec
ORGANISM: *Ircinia spinosula* (Porifera)
REFERENCE: 94

$C_{41}H_{60}O_2$ **2-Heptapyrenyl-1,4-benzoquinone**

MOL. WT.: 584
MELTING POINT: Oil
SPECTRAL DATA: UV, IR, PMR, Mass Spec
ORGANISM: *Ircinia spinosula* (Porifera)
REFERENCE: 94

C$_{41}$H$_{62}$O$_2$ **2-Heptapyrenyl-1,4-quinol**

MOL. WT.: 586
MELTING POINT: Oil
SPECTRAL DATA: UV, IR, PMR, Mass Spec
ORGANISM: *Ircinia spinosula* (Porifera)
REFERENCE: 94

C$_{46}$H$_{68}$O$_2$ **2-Octapyrenyl-1,4-benzoquinone**

MOL. WT.: 652
MELTING POINT: Oil
SPECTRAL DATA: UV, IR, PMR, Mass Spec
ORGANISM: *Ircinia spinosula* (Porifera)
REFERENCE: 94

C$_{46}$H$_{70}$O$_2$ **2-Octapyrenyl-1,4-quinol**

MOL. WT.: 654
MELTING POINT: Oil
SPECTRAL DATA: UV, IR, PMR, Mass Spec
ORGANISM: *Ircinia spinosula* (Porifera)
REFERENCE: 94

C$_{46}$H$_{70}$O$_3$ **25-Hydroxymethyl-2-octapyrenyl-1,4-quinol**

MOL. WT.: 670
MELTING POINT: Oil
SPECTRAL DATA: UV, IR, PMR, Mass Spec
ORGANISM: *Ircinia spinosula* (Porifera)
REFERENCE: 94

Chapter 14

Amino Acids

C₂H₇NO₃S   **Taurine (2-Aminoethanesulfonic acid)**

$$\overset{\displaystyle CH_2CH_2SO_3H}{\underset{\displaystyle NH_2}{|}}$$

MOL. WT.:   125
MELTING POINT: 328°C
SPECTRAL DATA: PMR
ORGANISM: *Calyx nicacensis, Geodia gigas* (Porifera),
             Turbo stenogyrus, and *Macrocallista*
             nimbosa (Mollusca)
REFERENCE: 10, 16, 339

C₂H₈NO₃P   **2-Aminoethyl-phosphonic acid**

$$H_2N-CH_2-CH_2-\overset{\displaystyle O}{\underset{\displaystyle OH}{\overset{\displaystyle \|}{P}}}-OH$$

MOL. WT.:   125
MELTING POINT: 280–281°C (dec.)
SPECTRAL DATA: IR
ORGANISM: *Anthopleura elegantissima* and *Metridium*
             dianthus (Coelenterata)
REFERENCE: 242, 346

C₃H₇N₃O₂   **Glycocyamine (Guanidoacetic acid)**

$$\underset{\displaystyle H_2N}{\overset{\displaystyle NH}{>}}C-NH-CH_2CO_2H$$

MOL. WT.:   117
MELTING POINT: 280–284°C; Hydrochloride, 200°C
             (dec.)
ORGANISM: *Anthopleura japonica* Verrill and
             Hippospongia equina (Coelenterata)
REFERENCE: 14, 283

145

C₃H₈NO₅P   α-Amino-β-phosphonopropionic acid

$$O=\overset{\underset{|}{OH}}{\underset{OH}{P}}-CH_2\overset{\underset{|}{NH_2}}{CH}-CO_2H$$

MOL. WT.: 169
ORGANISM: *Zoanthus sociatus* and *Tetrahymena*
            pyriformis (Protozoa)
REFERENCE: 240

C₃H₉NO₃S   Monomethyltaurine

$$\overset{\underset{|}{CH_2CH_2SO_3H}}{NHCH_3}$$

MOL. WT.: 139
MELTING POINT: 241–242°C
ORGANISM: *Calyx nicacensis* (Porifera)
REFERENCE: 16

C₃H₉N₃O₃S   Taurocyamine

$$\begin{array}{c} CH_2CH_2SO_3H \\ | \\ NH \\ | \\ HN{=}C \\ | \\ NH_2 \end{array}$$

MOL. WT.: 167
ORGANISM: *Calyx nicacensis* (Porifera)
REFERENCE: 16

C₃H₁₀NO₃P   2-Methylamino-ethylphosphonic acid

$$HN\overset{CH_3}{\underset{}{CH_2CH_2}}\overset{}{\underset{OH}{P}}{=}O$$

MOL. WT.: 139
MELTING POINT: 291°C (dec.)
ORGANISM: *Anthopleura xanthogrammica*
            (Coelenterata)
REFERENCE: 241

C₄H₉N₃O₂   β-Guanidinopropionic acid

$$\overset{HN}{\underset{H_2N}{>}}C{-}NH{-}CH_2{-}CH_2CO_2H$$

MOL. WT.: 131
MELTING POINT: 209–211°C
ORGANISM: *Anthopleura japonica* Verrill (Coelenterata)
REFERENCE: 283

C₄H₁₁NO₃S   Dimethyltaurine

$$\overset{\underset{|}{CH_2CH_2SO_3H}}{N(CH_3)_2}$$

MOL. WT.: 153
MELTING POINT: 315–316°C
ORGANISM: *Calyx nicacensis* (Porifera)
REFERENCE: 16

C$_5$H$_3$Br$_2$NO$_2$ **4,5-Dibromopyrrole-2-carboxylic acid**

MOL. WT.: 269
MELTING POINT: 148°C
SPECTRAL DATA: IR, Mass Spec
ORGANISM: *Agelas oroides* (Porifera)
REFERENCE: 147

C$_5$H$_9$NO$_4$ **Strombine**

MOL. WT.: 147
MELTING POINT: Hydrochloride, 131°C
ORGANISM: *Strombus gigas* (Mollusca)
REFERENCE: 354

C$_5$H$_{10}$N$_2$O$_5$S   **Arcamine**

MOL. WT.: 210
SPECTRAL DATA: Mass Spec
ORGANISM: *Arca zebra* (Mollusca)
REFERENCE: 354

C$_5$H$_{11}$NO$_2$

MOL. WT.: 117
MELTING POINT: ~310°C; HAuCl$_4$ complex, 224°C;
        Hydrobromide, 233°C (dec.)
ORGANISM: *Geodia gigas* (Porifera)
REFERENCE: 2

C$_5$H$_{11}$N$_3$O$_2$ **γ-Guanidino-butyric acid**

MOL. WT.: 145
MELTING POINT: Hydrochloride, 184°C
ORGANISM: *Anthopleura japonica* Verrill (Coelenterata)
REFERENCE: 283

$C_5H_{11}N_3O_3$ γ-Guanidino-β-hydroxybutyric acid

MOL. WT.: 161
MELTING POINT: 237°C
ORGANISM: *Anthopleura japonica* Verrill (Coelenterata)
REFERENCE: 283

$C_5H_{13}NO_3S$ Taurobetaine

MOL. WT.: 167
MELTING POINT: > 300°C
ORGANISM: *Geodia gigas* (Porifera)
REFERENCE: 5, 10

$C_6H_9N_3O_2$ Histidine

MOL. WT.: 155
MELTING POINT: 287°C (dec.); Dihydrochloride, 245°C
$[α]_D$: +40.2
ORGANISM: *Hippospongia equina* (Porifera)
REFERENCE: 14

$C_6H_{14}N_2O_2$ Lysine

MOL. WT.: 146
MELTING POINT: 224–225°C (dec.)
$[α]_D$: +14.6   SOLVENT: Aq
ORGANISM: *Hippospongia equina* (Porifera)
REFERENCE: 14

$C_9H_9BrClNO_3$ 3-Bromo-5-Chlorotyrosine

MOL. WT.: 295
ORGANISM: *Limulus polyphemus* L.
                (Arthropoda/Crustacea)
REFERENCE: 436

C$_9$H$_9$Br$_2$NO$_3$ 3,5-Dibromotyrosine

MOL. WT.: 339
MELTING POINT: 242–245°C
[α]$_D$: −5.5   SOLVENT: 1N HCl
SPECTRAL DATA: Mass Spec
ORGANISM: *Spongia officinalis obliqua* (Porifera) and
          Limulus polyphemus L. (Arthropoda/Crustacea)
REFERENCE: 1, 15, 282, 436

C$_9$H$_9$Cl$_2$NO$_3$ 3,5-Dichlorotyrosine

MOL. WT.: 250
ORGANISM: *Limulus polyphemus* L.
          (Arthropoda/Crustacea)
REFERENCE: 436

C$_9$H$_9$I$_2$NO$_3$ 3,5-Diiodotyrosine

MOL. WT.: 433
MELTING POINT: 204°C
[α]$_D$: +2.6   SOLVENT: Dil. HCl
ORGANISM: *Spongia officinalis obliqua* (Porifera)
REFERENCE: 1, 15, 282, 438

C$_9$H$_{10}$BrNO$_3$ 3-Bromotyrosine

MOL. WT.: 260
SPECTRAL DATA: Mass Spec
ORGANISM: *Limulus polyphemus* L.
          (Arthropoda/Crustacea)
REFERENCE: 436

C$_9$H$_{10}$ClNO$_3$ 3-Chlorotyrosine

MOL. WT.: 215
SPECTRAL DATA: Mass Spec
ORGANISM: *Limulus polyphemus* L.
          (Arthropoda/Crustacea)
REFERENCE: 436

$C_9H_{10}INO_3$ 3-Iodotyrosine

MOL. WT.: 307
ORGANISM: *Spongia officinalis obliqua* (Porifera)
REFERENCE: 282

$C_9H_{11}NO_3$ Tyrosine

MOL. WT.: 181
MELTING POINT: 342–344°C (dec.)
$[\alpha]_D$: -13.2 SOLVENT: 3N NaOH
ORGANISM: *Spongia officinalis obliqua* (Porifera)
REFERENCE: 282

$C_{18}H_{34}N_2O_{13}$ *O*-α-D-Glucopyranosyl-(1 → 2)- *O*-β-D-galactopyranosyloxy-(1 → 5)-L-Lysine

MOL. WT.: 486
$[\alpha]_D$: $+42$ SOLVENT: Aq
SPECTRAL DATA: PMR, Mass Spec
ORGANISM: *Hippospongia gossypina* (Porifera), *Metridium dianthus*
              (Coelenterata), and *Thyone briareus* (Echinodermata)
REFERENCE: 205, 221

Chapter 15

Amines and Nitrogen Heterocyclic Compounds

CH$_5$N$_3$ **Guanidine**

$$\underset{H_2N-C-NH_2}{\overset{NH}{\parallel}}$$

MOL. WT.: 59
MELTING POINT: ~50°C; Picrate, 333°C
ORGANISM: *Hippospongia equina* (Porifera)
REFERENCE: 2, 14

C$_2$H$_7$N   **Dimethylamine**

$(CH_3)_2NH$

MOL. WT.: 45
MELTING POINT: 7.4°C (b.p.)
ORGANISM: *Hippospongia equina* (Porifera)
REFERENCE: 14

C$_2$H$_7$N   **Ethylamine**

$CH_3CH_2NH_2$

MOL. WT.: 45
MELTING POINT: 16.6°C (b.p.); Hydrochloride, 108°C
ORGANISM: *Hippospongia equina* (Porifera)

C$_3$H$_9$N   **Propylamine**

$CH_3CH_2CH_2NH_2$

MOL. WT.: 59
MELTING POINT: 48.7°C (b.p.)
ORGANISM *Hippospongia equina* (Porifera)
REFERENCE: 14

C$_3$H$_9$N   Trimethylamine

$(CH_3)_3N$

MOL. WT.: 59
MELTING POINT: 3.5°C (b.p.); Hydrochloride, 275°C
ORGANISM: *Calyx nicacensis* (Porifera)
REFERENCE: 16

C$_4$H$_4$N$_2$O$_2$ Uracil

MOL. WT.: 112
MELTING POINT: 335°C
ORGANISM: *Cryptotethia crypta* (Porifera)
REFERENCE: 36

C$_4$H$_4$ClN$_3$O   5-Chlorocytosine

MOL. WT.: 145
SPECTRAL DATA: UV, Mass Spec
REFERENCE: 281

C$_4$H$_{12}$N$_2$ Putrescine

$H_2N—(CH_2)_4—NH_2$

MOL. WT.: 88
MELTING POINT: 27–28°C
ORGANISM: *Hippospongia equina* (Porifera)
REFERENCE: 14

C$_4$H$_{13}$NO   Tetramine

MOL. WT.: 91
MELTING POINT: 63°C
ORGANISM: *Actinia equina* (Mollusca)
REFERENCE: 3, 287

C$_5$H$_2$Br$_2$N$_2$

MOL. WT.: 250
MELTING POINT: 172–173°C
SPECTRAL DATA: IR, Mass Spec
ORGANISM: *Agelas oroides* (Porifera)
REFERENCE: 147

$C_5H_4Br_2N_2O$

MOL. WT.: 268
MELTING POINT: 164–166°C
SPECTRAL DATA: UV, IR, Mass Spec
ORGANISM: *Agelas oroides* (Porifera)
REFERENCE: 147

$C_5H_5N_5$ Adenine

MOL. WT.: 135
MELTING POINT: 360–365°C; Picrate, 277°C
ORGANISM: *Geodia gigas* (Porifera)
REFERENCE: 12

$C_5H_6N_2O_2$

MOL. WT.: 126
MELTING POINT: 222°C (dec.); Ethyl ester, 115–117°C
ORGANISM: *Hippospongia equina* (Porifera)
REFERENCE: 14

$C_5H_6N_2O_2$ Thymine

MOL. WT.: 126
MELTING POINT: 321°C
ORGANISM: *Cryptotethia crypta* (Porifera)
REFERENCE: 36

$C_5H_9N_3$ Histamine

MOL. WT.: 111
MELTING POINT: 83–84°C; Dipicrate, 241°C;
                 Monopicrate, 160–162°C;
                 Dihydrochloride, 244–246°C
ORGANISM: *Octopus apollyon, Octopus bimaculatus,*
                 Actinia equina (Mollusca), *Calliactis parasitica,*
                 Metridium senile (Coelenterata), *Geodia gigas* (Porifera),
                 and *Anemonia sulcata* (Coelenterata)
REFERENCE: 7, 13, 287

$C_5H_{11}NO$

$$CH_3\diagdown CHCH_2\overset{\overset{\displaystyle O}{\parallel}}{C}-NH_2$$
$$CH_3\diagup$$

MOL. WT.: 101
MELTING POINT: 132–134°C
SPECTRAL DATA: IR, PMR, Mass Spec
ORGANISM: *Thelepus setosus* (Annelida)
REFERENCE: 179

$C_5H_{11}NS_2$ Nereistoxin (4-Dimethylamino-1,2-dithiolane)

MOL. WT.: 149
BIOACTIVITY: Neurotoxin
MELTING POINT: 178–180°C
ORGANISM: *Lumbriconereis heteropoda* (Annelida)
REFERENCE: 319

$C_5H_{13}N$ Isoamylamine

$$CH_3\diagdown CHCH_2CH_2NH_2$$
$$CH_3\diagup$$

MOL. WT.: 87
MELTING POINT: 95°C (b.p.)
ORGANISM: *Hippospongia equina* (Porifera)
REFERENCE: 14

$C_5H_{14}NO_3P$ 2-Trimethylaminoethylphosphonic acid betaine

$$CH_3\overset{\overset{\displaystyle CH_3}{\mid}}{\underset{\underset{\displaystyle CH_3}{\mid}}{N^{\oplus}}}CH_2CH_2\overset{\overset{\displaystyle OH}{}}{\underset{\underset{\displaystyle O^{\ominus}}{}}{P}}=O$$

MOL. WT.: 167
MELTING POINT: 252°C (dec.)
ORGANISM: *Anthopleura xanthogrammica* (Coelenterata)
REFERENCE: 241

$C_5H_{14}N_4$ Agmatine

$$H_2N-(CH_2)_4-NH-\overset{\overset{\displaystyle }{}}{\underset{\underset{\displaystyle NH_2}{\mid}}{C}}=NH$$

MOL. WT.: 130
MELTING POINT: Picrate, 235–236°C; Sulfate, 229°C
ORGANISM: *Anthopleura japonica* Verrill (Coelenterata) and *Geodia gigas* (Porifera)
REFERENCE: 13, 283

C$_5$H$_{15}$NO$_2$ Choline

$$(CH_3)_3\overset{\oplus}{N}CH_2CH_2OH \cdot OH^{\ominus}$$

MOL. WT.: 121
ORGANISM: *Hippospongia equina* (Porifera)
REFERENCE: 14

C$_6$H$_5$Br$_2$NO$_2$

MOL. WT.: 283
MELTING POINT: 159–160°C
SPECTRAL DATA: Mass Spec
ORGANISM: *Agelas oroides* (Porifera)
REFERENCE: 147

C$_6$H$_6$N$_2$O$_2$ Imidazolyl acrylic acid (urocanic acid)

MOL. WT.: 138
MELTING POINT: 175–176°C; Dihydrate, 225°C
ORGANISM: *Hippospongia equina* (Porifera)
REFERENCE: 14

C$_6$H$_7$N$_5$ 1-Methyl-adenine (Spongopurine)

MOL. WT.: 149
MELTING POINT: Picrate, 255–257°C
SPECTRAL DATA: IR
ORGANISM: *Geodia gigas* (Porifera)
REFERENCE: 4, 8, 13

C$_6$H$_8$N$_2$O$_2$ 1,3-Dimethylimidazole-4-carboxylic acid betaine (Norzooanemonin)

MOL. WT.: 140
MELTING POINT: 260–263°C
SPECTRAL DATA: IR, PMR, Mass Spec
ORGANISM: *Pseudopterogorgia americana* Gmelin (Coelenterata)
REFERENCE: 430

$C_6H_8N_2O_2$

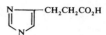

MOL. WT.: 140
MELTING POINT: 206–208°C; Anilide, 190–191°C
ORGANISM: *Hippospongia equina* (Porifera)
REFERENCE: 14

$C_6H_8N_2O_3$ Imidazolyl lactic acid

MOL. WT.: 156
MELTING POINT: 222°C; Ethyl ester, 118–119°C
ORGANISM: *Hippospongia equina* (Porifera)
REFERENCE: 14

$C_6H_{14}N_4O_3$ γ-Hydroxyarginine

MOL. WT.: 190
MELTING POINT: Hydrochloride, 190–191°C
$[\alpha]_D$: +6.3   SOLVENT: 2.5N HCl
ORGANISM: *Anthopleura japonica* Verrill (Coelenterata)
REFERENCE: 283

$C_6H_{16}N_6$ Arcaine

MOL. WT.: 172
MELTING POINT: Sulfate, 291°C (dec.); Picrate,
                 251–254°C (dec.)
ORGANISM: *Arca noar* (Mollusca)
REFERENCE: 348

$C_7H_7NO_2$ Homarine (*N*-Methyl-picolinic acid)

MOL. WT.: 137
MELTING POINT: Hydrochloride, 170–175°C
SPECTRAL DATA: UV
ORGANISM: *Calyx nicaensis* (Porifera)
REFERENCE: 16, 158

C₇H₇NO₂   Trigonelline (*N*-Methyl-nicotinic acid)

MOL. WT.: 137
MELTING POINT: 230–233°C; Hydrochloride,
                258–259°C; Picrate, 204–205°C
ORGANISM: *Calyx nicacensis* (Porifera)
REFERENCE: 16

**C₇H₉N₅O   2-Amino-6-hydroxy-7,9-dimethylpurine
betaine (Herbipoline)**

MOL. WT.: 179
MELTING POINT: 315°C; Picrate, 292–295°C
SPECTRAL DATA: IR
ORGANISM: *Geodia gigas* (Porifera)
REFERENCE: 6, 9, 11, 12, 53

**C₇H₁₀N₂O₂   1,3-Dimethyl-imidazole-4-acetic acid
betaine (Zooanemonine)**

MOL. WT.: 154
MELTING POINT: HAuCl₄ Complex Hydrochloride
ORGANISM: *Hippospongia equina* (Porifera)
REFERENCE: 9, 14

**C₇H₁₀N₂O₂   3,6-Dioxo-hexahydropyrrolo-[1,2-a]-
pyrazine**

MOL. WT.: 154
MELTING POINT: 216–218°C
SPECTRAL DATA: Mass Spec
ORGANISM: *Luidia clathrata* (Echinodermata)
REFERENCE: 340

C₇H₁₃N₃   Dimethyl histamine

MOL. WT.: 139
MELTING POINT: HAuCl₄ complex 198°C
ORGANISM: *Geodia gigas* (Porifera)
REFERENCE: 2

C₈H₁₁NO   **Tyramine**

HO—⟨benzene⟩—CH₂CH₂NH₂

MOL. WT.: 137
MELTING POINT: 164–165°C
REFERENCE: 122

C₈H₁₁NO₂   **Dopamine**

HO, HO—⟨benzene⟩—CH₂CH₂NH₂

MOL. WT.: 153
ORGANISM: *Octopus apollyon* and *Octopus bimaculatus*
            (Mollusca)
REFERENCE: 174

C₈H₁₁NO₂   **Octopamine**

HO—⟨benzene⟩—CH(OH)CH₂NH₂

MOL. WT.: 153
MELTING POINT: Hydrochloride, 177–179°
ORGANISM: *Octopus apollyon* and *Octopus bimaculatus*
            (Mollusca)
REFERENCE: 122, 174

C₈H₁₁NO₃   **Norepinephrine**

HO, HO—⟨benzene⟩—CH(OH)CH₂NH₂

MOL. WT.: 169
MELTING POINT: 216.5–218°C (dec.); Hydrochloride,
                 145.2–146.4°C
$[\alpha]_D$: −37.3   SOLVENT: 1M HCl
ORGANISM: *Octopus apollyon* (Mollusca), *Hydra littoralis* (Coelenterata),
            Octopus bimaculatus (Mollusca), and *Sycon (scypha) ciliatum*
            (Porifera)
REFERENCE: 277, 444

C₉H₇NO₂

MOL. WT.: 161
MELTING POINT: 300°C
SPECTRAL DATA: UV, IR, PMR, Mass Spec
ORGANISM: *Octopus dofleini* Martini (Mollusca)
REFERENCE: 391

$C_9H_8BrNO_4S_2$ 6-Bromo-2-methyl-thioindoxyl sulfate

MOL. WT.: 338
MELTING POINT: Ag Salt, 118–120°C
ORGANISM: *Dicathais orbita* Gmelin (Mollusca)
REFERENCE: 27

$C_9H_9Br_2NO_3$ (+)-Aeroplysinin-1

MOL. WT.: 339
MELTING POINT: 120°C; Diacetate, 114°C
$[\alpha]_D$: +186   SOLVENT: MeOH
SPECTRAL DATA: UV, IR, PMR, Mass Spec
ORGANISM: *Aplysina* (or *Verongia*) *aerophoba* (Porifera), and *Ianthella* sp. (Porifera)
REFERENCE: 106, 133, 134, 153

$C_9H_9Br_2NO_3$ (−)-Aeroplysinin-1

MOL. WT.: 339
MELTING POINT: 112–116°C
$[\alpha]_D$: −198   SOLVENT: An
SPECTRAL DATA: IR, PMR
ORGANISM: *Ianthella ardis* (Porifera)
REFERENCE: 106, 133, 134, 153

$C_9H_9NO_4$ 4-Hydroxyphenyl-pyruvic acid oxime

MOL. WT.: 195
SPECTRAL DATA: UV, PMR
ORGANISM: *Hymeniacidon sanguinea* (Porifera)
REFERENCE: 89

$C_9H_{12}ClN_3O_4$ 5-Chlorodeoxycytidine

MOL. WT.: 261
SPECTRAL DATA: Mass Spec
ORGANISM: Salmon Sperm (Chordata/Pisces)
REFERENCE: 281

$C_9H_{12}N_2O_6$ **1-β-D-Arabinofuranosyluracil (Spongouridine)**

MOL. WT.: 244
MELTING POINT: 226–228°C
SPECTRAL DATA: UV
ORGANISM: *Cryptotethia crypta* (Porifera)
REFERENCE: 36, 55

$C_9H_{13}NO_3$ **Epinephrine**

MOL. WT.: 183
MELTING POINT: 211–212°C
$[\alpha]_D$: −53.5   SOLVENT: 0.5N HCl
ORGANISM: *Sycon* (or *Scypha*) *ciliatum* (Porifera), *Octopus apollyon*, *Octopus bimaculatus* (Mollusca), and *Hydra littoralis* (Coelenterata)
REFERENCE: 277, 444

$C_9H_{15}N_3O_2$ **Hercynine**

MOL. WT.: 197
MELTING POINT: 224–228°C (dec.); HAuCl₄ complex, 184°C; Dipicrate, 213–214°C
ORGANISM: *Hippospongia equina* (Porifera)
REFERENCE: 14

$C_9H_{18}N_4O_4$ **Octopine**

MOL. WT.: 246
MELTING POINT: 281–282°C; Picrate, 225°C
$[\alpha]_D$: +20.94   SOLVENT: Aq
REFERENCE: 18

$C_{10}H_7NO_4$ **3,4-Dihydroxyquinoline-2-carboxylic acid**

MOL. WT.: 205
MELTING POINT: 253–254°C (dec.)
SPECTRAL DATA: UV, IR, Mass Spec
ORGANISM: *Aplysina* (or *Verongia*) *aerophoba* (Porifera)
REFERENCE: 126

$C_{10}H_{10}Br_2N_2$ 3-(2-Aminoethyl)-5,6-dibromoindole

MOL. WT.: 318
MELTING POINT: 110–120°C
SPECTRAL DATA: UV, PMR, Mass Spec
ORGANISM: *Polyfibrospongia maynardii* Hyatt (Porifera)
REFERENCE: 424

$C_{10}H_{10}N_6$ Parazoanthoxanthin A

MOL. WT.: 214
MELTING POINT: > 310
SPECTRAL DATA: PMR
ORGANISM: *Parazoanthus axinellae* (Coelenterata)
REFERENCE: 70

$C_{10}H_{12}N_2$ Anabaseine[2-(3-pyridyl)-3,4,5,6-tetrahydropyridine]

MOL. WT.: 160
BIOACTIVITY: Neurotoxin
MELTING POINT: Picrate, 172–175°C
SPECTRAL DATA: UV, PMR, Mass Spec
ORGANISM: *Paranemertes peregrina* Coe (Nemertinea)
REFERENCE: 227

$C_{10}H_{12}N_2O$ Serotonin (5-Hydroxytryptamine)

MOL. WT.: 176
BIOACTIVITY: Vasoconstrictor
MELTING POINT: Hydrochloride, 167–168°C
ORGANISM: *Octopus apollyon, Octopus bimaculatus,*
           Octopus vulgaris (Mollusca), *Physalia* sp.,
           Hydra oligactis, Hydra littoralis (Coelenterata),
           and *Sycon* (or *Scypha*) *ciliatum* (Porifera)
REFERENCE: 122, 243, 277

$C_{10}H_{14}N_2O_6$ 1-β-D-Arabinosylthymine (Spongothymidine)

MOL. WT.:   258

MELTING POINT: 246–247°C; Tribenzoate, 190–191°C;
                 Tri-*p*-bromobenzoate, 251–252°C

$[\alpha]_D$:   +80; +92   SOLVENT: 8% NaOH; Py

ORGANISM: *Cryptotethia crypta* (Porifera)

REFERENCE: 36, 37, 38

$C_{10}H_{17}N_7O_3 \cdot 2HCl$ Saxitoxin

MOL. WT.:   283

MELTING POINT: Dihydrochloride

$[\alpha]_D$:   +130

SPECTRAL DATA: PMR

ORGANISM: *Gonyaulaux catenella* and *Gonyaulaux tamarensis* (Protozoa)

REFERENCES: 314, 358, 359, 371, 443

$C_{11}H_{11}Br_2N_5O$ Dibromophakellin

MOL. WT.:   389

MELTING POINT: 237–245°C (dec.); Monoacetate, 240–250°C

$[\alpha]_D$:   −203

SPECTRAL DATA: UV, IR, Mass Spec

ORGANISM: *Phakellia flabellata* (Porifera)

REFERENCE: 373

$C_{11}H_{11}Br_2N_5O$ Oroidin

MOL. WT.:   389

MELTING POINT: *N*-Acetate, 256–258°C; Dihydro-*N*-Acetate, 244–247°C

SPECTRAL DATA: UV, IR

ORGANISM: *Agelas oroides* (Porifera)

REFERENCE: 147

$C_{11}H_{12}BrN_5O$ 4-Bromophakellin

MOL. WT.: 310
MELTING POINT: 170–180°C (dec.)
ORGANISM: *Phakellia flabellata* (Porifera)
REFERENCE: 373

$C_{11}H_{12}Br_2N_2$ 2-*N*-Methylamino-3-(ethyl)-indole

MOL. WT.: 332
BIOACTIVITY: Antibiotic
MELTING POINT: 132–134°C
SPECTRAL DATA: UV, PMR, Mass Spec
ORGANISM: *Polyfibrospongia maynardii* Hyatt (Porifera)
REFERENCE: 424

$C_{11}H_{12}N_6$ 3-Norpseudozoanthoxanthin

MOL. WT.: 228
MELTING POINT: 230°C (dec.)
SPECTRAL DATA: UV, PMR, Mass Spec
ORGANISM: *Epizoanthus arenaceus*
              (Arthropoda/Crustacea)
REFERENCE: 71

$C_{11}H_{15}N_5O_5$ Spongosine

MOL. WT.: 297
MELTING POINT: 192–193°C
$[\alpha]_D$: −42.5   SOLVENT: 8% NaOH
ORGANISM: *Cryptotethia crypta* (Porifera)
REFERENCE: 35, 38, 45

$C_{11}H_{17}N_3O_8$ Tetrodotoxin

MOL. WT.: 319
MELTING POINT: >220°C; Picrate, >200°C
$[\alpha]_D$: −8.64   SOLVENT: Dil. HOAc
SPECTRAL DATA: UV
ORGANISM: *Spheroides rubripes* (Chordata/Pisces)
REFERENCE: 161

$C_{11}H_{19}N_3O_3$ **Murexine Urocanylcholine**

$$N\text{---}CH\text{=}CHCO_2CH_2CH_2\overset{\oplus}{N}(CH_3)_3\overset{\ominus}{O}H$$

MOL. WT.: 241
MELTING POINT: Picrate, 218–221°C
ORGANISM: *Murex trunculus, Murex grandaris*, and
           Murex erinaceus (Mollusca)
REFERENCE: 121

$C_{12}H_{14}N_6$ **Parazoanthoxanthin D**

MOL. WT.: 242
MELTING POINT: 303–304°C
SPECTRAL DATA: UV, IR, Mass Spec
ORGANISM: *Parazoanthus axinellae* (Coelenterata)
REFERENCE: 70

$C_{12}H_{14}N_6$ **Pseudozoanthoxanthin**

MOL. WT.: 242
MELTING POINT: > 310°C
SPECTRAL DATA: UV, PMR, Mass Spec
ORGANISM: *Epizoanthus arenaceus*
           (Arthropoda/Crustacea)
REFERENCE: 71

$C_{13}H_{12}Br_2N_2O_5$ **LL-PAA216**

MOL. WT.: 452
MELTING POINT: 222–225°C
$[\alpha]_D$: +8.9   SOLVENT: MeOH
SPECTRAL DATA: UV, IR, PMR, Mass Spec
ORGANISM: *Verongia lacunosa* (Porifera)
REFERENCE: 49

$C_{13}H_{16}N_6$ **Epizoanthoxanthin A**

MOL. WT.: 256
MELTING POINT: 191–192°C
SPECTRAL DATA: UV, PMR
ORGANISM: *Epizoanthus arenaceus*
           (Arthropoda/Crustacea)
REFERENCE: 71

$C_{13}H_{16}N_6$ **Paragracine**

MOL. WT.: 256
MELTING POINT: 258–262°C (dec.); Acetate, 233–235°C
SPECTRAL DATA: UV, PMR, Mass Spec
ORGANISM: *Parazoanthus gracilis* Lwowsky
     (Coelenterata)
REFERENCE: 250

$C_{13}H_{16}N_6$ **Zoanthoxanthin (2-Amino-3,4-
     dimethyl-6-dimethylamino-3H-
     1,3,5,7-tetra-azacyclopent[f]azulene)**

MOL. WT.: 256
MELTING POINT: 275–276°C
SPECTRAL DATA: UV, IR, PMR, Mass Spec
ORGANISM: *Parazoanthus axinellae* (Coelenterata)
REFERENCE: 68, 69

$C_{14}H_{14}N_4O$ **Aplysinopsin**

MOL. WT.: 254
MELTING POINT: 232–233°C; Diacetate, 217–220°C
SPECTRAL DATA: UV, IR, PMR, Mass Spec
ORGANISM: *Thorecta* sp. and *Verongia spengelii* (Porifera)
REFERENCE: 222

$C_{14}H_{18}N_6$ **Epizoanthoxanthin B**

MOL. WT.: 270
MELTING POINT: Amph.
SPECTRAL DATA: UV, PMR, Mass Spec
ORGANISM: *Epizoanthus arenaceus*
     (Arthropoda/Crustacea)
REFERENCE: 71

$C_{15}H_{15}NO$ Navenone A

MOL. WT.:   225
MELTING POINT: 144–145°C
SPECTRAL DATA: UV, IR, PMR, Mass Spec
ORGANISM: *Navanax inermis* (Cooper) (Mollusca)
REFERENCE: 392

$C_{16}H_8Br_2N_2O_2$ 6,6′-Dibromo-indigotin

MOL. WT.:   420
MELTING POINT: *N,N′*-Diacetyl 306°C
ORGANISM: *Dicathais orbita* Gmelin (Mollusca)
REFERENCE: 27

$C_{16}H_{22}Cl_3NO_4$ Dysidin

MOL. WT.:   397
MELTING POINT: 127–129°C
$[\alpha]_D$:   +141   SOLVENT: Chf
SPECTRAL DATA: UV, IR, PMR, Mass Spec
ORGANISM: *Dysidea herbacea* (Porifera)
REFERENCE: 184

$C_{16}H_{25}N$ Acanthellin-1

MOL. WT.:   231
BIOACTIVITY: Antibacterial
MELTING POINT: Oil
$[\alpha]_D$:   −41.2
SPECTRAL DATA: IR, PMR, Mass Spec
ORGANISM: *Acanthella acuta* (Platyhelminthes)
REFERENCE: 296

$C_{16}H_{25}N$ Acanthellin-2

MOL. WT.:   231
MELTING POINT: Oil
$[\alpha]_D$:   −24.1
SPECTRAL DATA: IR, Mass Spec
ORGANISM: *Acanthella acuta* (Platyhelminthes)
REFERENCE: 296

$C_{16}H_{25}N$ Axisonitrile-1

MOL. WT.: 231
MELTING POINT: 43–45°C
[α]_D: +22.6   SOLVENT: Chf
SPECTRAL DATA: IR, PMR, Mass Spec
ORGANISM: *Axinella cannabina* (Porifera)
REFERENCE: 65

$C_{16}H_{25}N$ Axisonitrile-2

MOL. WT.: 231
MELTING POINT: Oil
[α]_D: +29   SOLVENT: Chf
SPECTRAL DATA: IR, PMR, Mass Spec
ORGANISM: *Axinella cannabina* (Porifera)
REFERENCE: 129

$C_{16}H_{25}N$ 9-Isocyanopupukeanane

MOL. WT.: 231
MELTING POINT: Oil
[α]_D: −9   SOLVENT: Cte
SPECTRAL DATA: IR, PMR, Mass Spec
ORGANISM: *Phyllidia varicosa* (Mollusca) and
          Hymeniacidon sp. (Porifera)
REFERENCE: 60

$C_{16}H_{25}N$

MOL. WT.: 231
MELTING POINT: 40–42°C
[α]_D: −75   SOLVENT: Cte
SPECTRAL DATA: IR, PMR
ORGANISM: *Halichondria* sp. (Porifera)
REFERENCE: 47, 57, 58

$C_{16}H_{25}NS$ Axisothiocyanate-1

MOL. WT.: 263
MELTING POINT: Oil
$[\alpha]_D$: +5.9   SOLVENT: Chf
SPECTRAL DATA: IR, PMR, Mass Spec
ORGANISM: *Axinella cannabina* (Porifera)
REFERENCE: 65

$C_{16}H_{25}NS$ Axisothiocyanate-2

MOL. WT.: 263
MELTING POINT: Oil
$[\alpha]_D$: +12.8
SPECTRAL DATA: IR, PMR, Mass Spec
ORGANISM: *Axinella cannabina* (Porifera)
REFERENCE: 128

$C_{16}H_{25}NS$

MOL. WT.: 263
MELTING POINT: Oil
$[\alpha]_D$: −63   SOLVENT: Cte
SPECTRAL DATA: UV, IR
ORGANISM: *Halichondria* sp. (Porifera)
REFERENCE: 57, 58, 59

$C_{16}H_{27}NO$ Axamide-1

MOL. WT.: 249
MELTING POINT: Oil
$[\alpha]_D$: +10
SPECTRAL DATA: IR, PMR, Mass Spec
ORGANISM: *Axinella cannabina* (Porifera)
REFERENCE: 128

$C_{16}H_{27}NO$ Axamide-2

MOL. WT.: 249
MELTING POINT: Oil
$[\alpha]_D$: 37.5
SPECTRAL DATA: IR, PMR, Mass Spec
ORGANISM: *Axinella cannabina* (Porifera)
REFERENCE: 128

$C_{16}H_{27}NO$

MOL. WT.: 249
$[\alpha]_D$: -50 SOLVENT: Cte
SPECTRAL DATA: IR, PMR, Mass Spec
ORGANISM: *Halichondria* sp. (Porifera)
REFERENCE: 57, 58, 59

$C_{17}H_{15}N_3O$ Aequorin

MOL. WT.: 277
MELTING POINT: 217–219°C
SPECTRAL DATA: UV, PMR, Mass Spec
ORGANISM: *Aequorea* sp. (Coelenterata)
REFERENCE: 234

$C_{20}H_{17}N_3O_9$ Xanthommatin

MOL. WT.: 443
SPECTRAL DATA: UV
ORGANISM: *Octopus vulgaris, Sepia officinalis, Loligo vulgaris,* and *Homarus gammarus* (Mollusca)
REFERENCE: 53, 61

$C_{20}H_{19}N_3O_9$ Dihydroxanthommatin

MOL. WT.: 445
MELTING POINT: $> 350°C$
SPECTRAL DATA: UV, IR
ORGANISM: *Octopus vulgaris, Sepia officinalis, Loligo vulgaris,* and *Homarus gammarus* (Mollusca)
REFERENCE: 48, 61

$C_{21}H_{28}N_7O$ Oxyluciferin

MOL. WT.: 394
MELTING POINT: 140–148°C
ORGANISM: *Cypridina hilgendorfii* (Arthropoda/Crustacea)
REFERENCE: 387

$C_{21}H_{33}N$ **3-Isocyano-3,7,11,15-tetramethyl-
1,6,10,14-hexadecatetraene**

MOL. WT.: 299
MELTING POINT: Oil
$[\alpha]_D$: +15   SOLVENT: Cte
SPECTRAL DATA: UV, IR, PMR, Mass Spec
ORGANISM: *Halichondria* sp. (Porifera)
REFERENCE: 58, 59

$C_{21}H_{33}NS$ **3-Isothiocyano-3,7-11,15-tetramethyl-
1,6,10,14-hexadecatetraene**

MOL. WT.: 331
ORGANISM: *Halichondria* sp. (Porifera)
REFERENCE: 58, 59

$C_{21}H_{35}NO$ **3,7,11,15-Tetramethyl-1,6,10,14-
hexadecatetraene-3-formamide**

MOL. WT.: 317
MELTING POINT: Oil
SPECTRAL DATA: IR, Mass Spec
ORGANISM: *Halichondria* sp. (Porifera)
REFERENCE: 58, 59

$C_{22}H_{27}N_7O$ **Luciferin**

MOL. WT.: 405
MELTING POINT: 182–195°C
ORGANISM: *Cypridina hilgendorfii*
                 (Arthropoda/Crustacea)
REFERENCE: 387

$C_{23}H_{46}ClNO_4$ Pahutoxin

$$\underset{\substack{| \\ CH_3-(CH_2)_{12}-CH-CH_2-COOCH_2CH_2-\overset{\oplus}{N}(CH_3)_3}}{\overset{OCOCH_3}{}}$$
$$Cl^{\ominus}$$

MOL. WT.:   436
BIOACTIVITY: Haemolytic
MELTING POINT: 74–75°C
$[\alpha]_D$:   +3.05   SOLVENT: Me
ORGANISM: *Ostracion lentiginosus* (Chordata/Pisces)
REFERENCE: 51

$C_{24}H_{26}Br_4N_4O_8$ Aerothionin

MOL. WT.:   818
MELTING POINT: 134–137°C; Diacetate, 206–208°C
$[\alpha]_D$:   +252   SOLVENT: An
SPECTRAL DATA: UV, IR, PMR, Mass Spec
ORGANISM: *Verongia thiona* and *Aplysina* (or *Verongia*) *aerophoba*
              (Porifera)
REFERENCE: 135, 305

$C_{25}H_{26}BrN_5O_{13}$ Surugatoxin

MOL. WT.:   684
MELTING POINT: >300°C
SPECTRAL DATA: UV, IR
ORGANISM: *Babylonia japonica* (Mollusca)
REFERENCE: 251

$C_{25}H_{28}Br_4N_4O_8$ Homoaerothionin

MOL. WT.: 832
MELTING POINT: Amph. Solid Diacetate, 166–167°C
SPECTRAL DATA: PMR
ORGANISM: *Verongia thiona* and *Aplysina* (or *Verongia*) *aerophoba*
             (Porifera)
REFERENCE: 132, 305

$C_{26}H_{40}ClN_5$ Agelasine

MOL. WT.: 458
MELTING POINT: 197–200°C (dec.)
SPECTRAL DATA: UV, IR, PMR, Mass Spec
ORGANISM: *Agelas dispar* Duchassaing and Michelotti (Porifera)
REFERENCE: 109

$C_{33}H_{36}N_4O_6$ Biliverdin IX,α

MOL. WT.: 584
SPECTRAL DATA: UV, Mass Spec
ORGANISM: *Heliopora coerulea* Pall. (Coelenterata)
REFERENCE: 351

$C_{45}H_{59}N_{11}O_{11}$

pGlu-Leu-Asn-Phe-Ser-Pro-Gly-Trp-NH$_2$

MOL. WT.: 929
ORGANISM: *Pandalus borealis* (Arthropoda/Crustacea)
REFERENCE: 146

$C_{54}H_{85}N_{13}O_{15}S$ Eledoisin

pGlu-Pro-Ser-Lys-Asp-Ala-Phe-Ile-Gly-Leu-Met-NH$_2$

(OH above Ser)

MOL. WT.: 1187
BIOACTIVITY: Hypotensive, 3–30 mg/kg
MELTING POINT: 230°C
$[\alpha]_D$: -44 SOLVENT: 95% HOAc
ORGANISM: *Eledone moschata* and *Eledone aldrovandi* (Mollusca)
REFERENCE: 120

$C_{207}H_{398}N_{57}O_{102}$ Anthopleurin-A

Asp-Asp-Asp-Asp-Thr-Thr-Thr-Ser-Ser-
Ser-Ser-Ser-Ser-Glu-Pro-Pro-Pro-Pro-
Gly-Gly-Gly-Gly-Gly-Gly-Gly-Gly-Ala-
Cys-Cys-Cys-Cys-Cys-Cys-Val-Val-Ile-
Leu-Leu-Leu-Leu-Tyr-Lys-Lys-His-His-
Arg-Trp-Trp-Tyr-(NH$_3$)$_3$

MOL. WT.: 5086
BIOACTIVITY: Positive Inotropic Effect
ORGANISM: *Anthopleura xanthogrammica* (Brandt)
           (Coelenterata)
REFERENCE: 315

22,000–24,000   Protein

BIOACTIVITY: Toxin
ORGANISM: *Octopus dofleini* Martini (Mollusca)
REFERENCE: 399

Subject Index

Section A

A. HIGHER PLANTS

Acanthospermum glabratum (DC.) Wild, 22

Baccharis megapotamica Spreng, 13

Coriolus versicolor, 25

Coronilla varia L. (var. *penngift*), 17, 21, 23

Gnidia glaucus Fres., 14

Gnidia latifolia Gilg., 14, 15

Gnidia subcordata Meissn. Engl., 15

Helenium microcephalum, 9, 10, 11

Isodon japonicus, 10, 11, 12

Isodon trichocarpus, 10, 11, 12

Jacaranda caucana Pittier, 21

Jatropha macrorhiza Benth., 10

Juncus roemerianus, 23

Lychnophora affinis Gardn., 22, 23, 24

Ophiorrhiza mungos Linn., 27

Penstemon deutus Dougl. ex Lindl., 11

Phyllanthus brasiliensis (Muell.), 12, 14

Polygala macradenia Gray, 19

Quassia amara L., 12

Rhamnus frangula L., 21

Samadera indica, 9, 11

Sargassum thunbergii, 25

Stemodia maritima, 10

Tithonia tagitiflora Desf., 24

Uvaria chamae, 19, 20, 22, 24, 25

Uvaria cucuminata Oliv., 19, 20

Vauquelinia corymbosa Correa, 13

B. HIGHER PLANT COMPONENTS

Aloe emodin, 21

Baccharin, 13

Berbamine, 29

Betulinic acid, 13

Camptothecin, 27

Cepharanoline, 28

Cepharanthine, 29

Chamanetin, 24

Cycleanine, 30

Daphnoretin, 23

Dauricine, 31

4'-Demethyldeoxypodo-phyllotoxin, 19

Dichamanetin, 25

3,5-Dihydroxy-4',7-dimethoxyflavone, 22

3',5-Dihydroxy-4',5',7,8-tetramethoxyflavone, 24

4',5-Dihydroxy-3',7,8-trimethoxyflavone, 23

3,6-Dimethoxy-4',5,7-trihydroxyflavone, 22

Diuvaretin, 20

Enmein, 10

Epistephanine, 29

Fangchinoline, 29

Gnidiglaucin, 14

Gnidilatidin, 14

Gnidilatidin 20-palmitate, 15

Gnidilatin, 14

Gnidilatin 20-palmitate, 15

Gnidimacrin, 15

Gnidimacrin 20-palmitate, 15

5-Hydroxy-3',4',7,8-tetramethoxyflavone, 24

5-Hydroxy-3',4',7-trimethoxyflavone, 23

Hypoepistephanine, 28

Hyrcanoside, 17

Insularine dimethiodide, 32

Isochamanetin, 25

Isoliensinine dihydrochloride, 30

Isouvaretin, 19

Jacaranone, 21

Jatrophatrione, 10

Juncusol, 23

10-Methoxycamptothecin, 27

0-Methyldauricine, 31

0-Methylthalicberine, 31

Mexicanin-E, 9

Microhelenin-A, 9

Microhelenin-B, 11

Microhelenin-C, 10

Oridonin, 11

Oxyacanthine dimethiodide, 32

Penstemide, 11

Phyllanthocin, 12

Phyllanthoside, 14

Pinocembrin, 22

Pinostrobin, 22

Polysaccharide, 25
Polysaccharide F-1, 25
Polysaccharide F-2, 25
Quassimarin, 12
Samaderin A, 9
Samaderin E, 11
Simalikalactone D, 12
Stebisimine, 29
Stemolide, 10
Tagitinin F, 24
Tetraandrine dimethiodide, 32
Tetramethylmagnolamine, 33
Thalicberine, 30
Trichokaurin, 12
Trilobine, 28
Umbelliferone, 21
Ursolic acid, 13
Uvaol, 13
Uvaretin, 19, 20

C. FUNGI AND OTHER LOWER PLANTS

Chaetomium globosum, 37, 38
Cladonia leptoclada des. Abb., 35
Fomes fomentarius, 39
Penicillium aurantio-virens Biourge, 37
Penicillium vermiculatum Dangeard, 36
Phomopsis sp., 37
Streptomyces achromogenes var. *tomaymyceticus*, 36
Streptomyces nogalater var. *nogalater* sp.n., 39
Streptomyces paulus Dietz. sp.n., 38
Streptomyces refuineus var. *thermotolerans*, 36
Streptomyces sp., 39
Streptomyces sviceus, 35
Streptosporangium pseudovulgare, 39
Streptosporangium sibiricum, 37

D. FUNGI AND OTHER LOWER PLANT COMPONENTS

Anthramycin, 36
Chaetoglobosin C, 37

Chaetoglobosin D, 38
Chaetoglobosin E, 38
Chaetoglobosin F, 38
Cytochalasin H, 37
Kodo-cytochalasin-1, 37
Neothramycin A, 39
Neothramycin B, 39
Nogalamycin, 39
Polysaccharide, unknown, 39
Primocarcin, 35
Sibiromycin, 37
Sporamycin, 39
Tomaymycin, 46
Usnic acid, 35
Vermiculine, 36

E. MARINE INVERTEBRATES AND OTHER LOWER ANIMALS

Dolabella ecaudata, 41
Vespula pensylvanica, 41

F. MARINE INVERTEBRATE AND OTHER LOWER ANIMAL BIOSYNTHETIC PRODUCTS

Loliolide, 41
Oleic acid, 41
Palmitoleic acid, 41

G. MARINE VERTEBRATES AND OTHER HIGHER ANIMALS

Naja naja atra, 43
Sphyrna lewini, 43, 44
Strongylocentrotus drobachiensis, 44

H. MARINE VERTEBRATE AND OTHER HIGHER ANIMAL BIOSYNTHETIC PRODUCTS

Prostaglandin E$_1$, 43
Sphyrnastatin 1, 43
Sphyrnastatin 2, 44
Strongylostatin 1, 44
Strongylostatin 2, 44

Section B

A. MARINE ANIMALS

Acanthaster planci Linn., 68, 71, 75, 76, 82, 85, 133

Acanthella acuta, 166
Actinia equina, 152, 153
Actinopyga agassizi, 111, 112, 115, 116, 117, 118, 125, 126
Aequorea sp., 169
Agelas dispar Duchassaing and Michelotti, 172
Agelas oroides, 147, 152, 153, 155, 162
Alcyonarian nephtea, 77
Amphidinium operculatum, 119
Anemonia sulcata, 153
Anthocidaris cassispina, 129
Anthopleura elegantissima, 145
Anthopleura japonica Verrill, 145, 146, 147, 148, 154, 156
Anthopleura xanthogrammica, 119, 146, 154, 173
Aplysia californica, 87, 92
Aplysia dactylomela, 90, 91, 95
Aplysia depilans, 98, 101
Aplysia kurodai, 90, 102
Aplysina (or *Verongia*) *aerophoba*, 79, 80, 87, 159, 160, 171, 172
Arca noar, 156
Arca zebra, 147
Arenicola marina, 141
Artemia salina L., 72
Asterias amurensis Lutkin, 65, 66, 69, 70, 72, 73, 74, 75
Asterias rubens, 120
Asterina pectinifera, 72
Axinella cannabina, 68, 72, 74, 96, 167, 168
Axinella polypoides, 67, 72, 76
Axinella verrucosa, 73, 77, 81
Babylonia japonica, 171
Balanoglossus biminiensis, 127
Balanus glandula, 70, 72
Bohadschia koellikeri, 112, 113, 115, 116
Cachonina niei, 119
Cacospongia mollior, 110
Cacospongia scalaris, 110

Calliactis parasitica, 153
Callinectes sapidus, 71, 75
Calyx nicaaensis, 66, 68
Calyx nicacensis, 126, 145, 146, 152, 156, 157
Calyx nicaensis, 77
Capnella imbricata, 96
Cardium corbis, 75
Certonardoa semiregularis, 72
Chionoecetes opilio, 72
Chiton tuberculatus L., 72
Chondrilla nucula Schmidt, 74, 78
Chondrilla sp., 107
Chrysophrys major Temminck, 119, 120, 121, 122, 123
Cliona celata, 66, 72
Comantheria perplexa, 135, 136, 138
Comanthus bennetti, 136, 137, 140
Comanthus parvicirrus timorensis J. Müller, 138, 139, 140
Comatula cratera Clark, 139, 140
Comatula pectinata, Linn., 139, 140
Condylactis gigantea, 61, 62
Crassius auratus, 121
Cryptotethia crypta, 150, 153, 160, 162, 163
Ctenodiseus crispatus Retzius, 72
Cypridina hilgendorfii, 169, 170
Diadema antillarum, 134
Dicathais orbita Gmelin, 159, 166
Disidea avora, 103, 104
Disidea herbacea, 130, 132
Disidea pallescens, 88, 89, 91, 92, 93, 104
Distolasterias sticantha, 72
Dysidea herbacea, 166
Echinometra oblonga, 132
Echinothrix calamaris Pallis, 128, 129, 130, 131, 132, 133, 134, 135
Echinothrix diadema Linn., 128, 129, 130, 131, 132, 133, 134, 135

Echinus esculentus, 129
Eledone aldrovandi, 173
Eledone moschata, 173
Epizoanthus arenaceus, 163, 164, 165
Eugorgia ampla, 72
Eunicea asperula, 101
Eunicea mammosa Lamouroux, 94, 95, 99
Eunicea tourneforti, 101
Eunicella stricta, 111
Galeocerdo arcticus, 73
Geodia gigas, 126, 145, 147, 148, 153, 154, 155, 157
Gonyaulaux catenella, 162
Gonyaulaux tamarensis, 162
Gorgonia flabellum L., 78
Gorgonia ventalina, 89
Gorgonia ventibna L., 78
Gyrinidae, 88
Halichondria panicea, 97
Halichondria sp., 167, 168, 169, 170
Haliclona permollis, 66, 74, 75, 78, 79
Haliclona sp., 66, 73, 74, 75, 78, 79
Halla parthenopeia, 135
Halocynthia papillosa, 118, 121
Haloderima grisea L., 113
Heliopora coerulea Pall., 172
Heteronema erecta, 77
Hippospongia communis, 102, 103, 105
Hippospongia equina, 145, 148, 151, 152, 153, 154, 155, 156, 157, 160
Hippospongia gossypina, 150
Holothuria polii, 111, 112, 113, 115, 116
Holothuria tabulosa, 125, 126
Homarus gammarus, 169
Hydra littoralis, 158, 160, 161
Hydra oligactis, 161
Hymeniacidon perleve, 67, 72, 77
Hymeniacidon sanguinea, 159

Hymeniacidon sanguineum Grant, 122
Hymeniacidon sp., 167
Ianthella ardis, 159
Ianthella sp., 87, 159
Ircinia fasciculata, 108
Ircinia muscarum, 110
Ircinia oros, 104, 108
Ircinia spinosula, 109, 112, 114, 117, 118, 142, 143
Ircinia variabilis Schmidt, 109
Jasus lalandei, 71
Lemnalia africana, 96
Limulus polyphemus L., 148, 149
Lissodendoryx noxiosa, 66, 69, 73, 74, 75, 78, 79, 80
Litophyton viridis, 76, 81, 101
Lobophytum cristagalli von Marenzeller, 97
Lobophytum sp., 105
Loligo vulgaris, 169
Luidia clathrata, 157
Lumbriconereis heteropoda, 154
Lysastrosoma anthostictha, 72
Lytechinus variegatus, 72
Macrocallista nimbosa, 145
Madrepora cervicornis, 70
Marthasterias glacialis, 68, 70
Meandra areolata, 72
Metridium dianthus, 145, 150
Metridium senile, 153
Microciona toxystila, 92, 93
Modiolus demissus, 75
Murex erinaceus, 164
Murex grandaris, 164
Murex trunculus, 164
Muricea appressa, 72
Navanax inermis (Cooper), 61, 166
Nephthea sp., 101, 106
Octopus apollyon, 153, 158, 160, 161
Octopus bimaculatus, 153, 158, 160, 161
Octopus dofleini Martini, 158, 173
Octopus vulgaris, 161, 169

Oligoceras hemorrhages, 92
Ophiocoma erinaceus, 132, 133, 134
Ophiocoma insularia, 132, 133, 134
Ostracion lentiginosus, 171
Palythoa mammilosa, 63
Palythoa sp., 75
Palythoa tuberculara, 82
Pandalus borealis, 172
Paracentrotus lividus Lam., 114, 123, 129, 131
Paralithodes sp., 72
Paranemertes peregrina Coe, 161
Parazoanthus axinellae, 161, 164, 165
Parazoanthus gracilis Lwowsky, 165
Pecten caurinus, 75
Pecten maximus, 121
Periphylla periphylla, 80
Phakellia flabellata, 162, 163
Phoronopsis viridis Hilton, 127
Phyllidia varicosa, 167
Physalia sp., 161
Pisaster ochraceus, 74
Placopecten magellanicus Gmelin, 67, 69
Pleraplysilla spinifera, 88, 90, 91, 92, 97
Plexaura homomalla, 99, 100, 105, 107
Plexaura sp., 72
Polycheira rufescens, 130
Polyfibrospongia maynardii Hyatt, 161, 163
Polypodium vulgare L., 71
Psammechinus miliaris Gmelin, 129
Pseudoplexaura crassa, 106
Pseudoplexaura porosa, 75, 79, 81, 106
Pseudoplexaura wagenaari, 106
Pseudopotamilla occelata Moore, 70, 72
Pseudopterogorgia americana Gmelin, 83, 94, 95, 155
Pterogorgia anceps Pallas, 106

Pterogorgia quadalupensis, 109
Ptilometra australis Wilton, 137, 138
Ptilosarcus gurneyi (Gray), 67, 107, 110
Reniera fulva, 62, 63
Reniera japonica, 119, 120, 122
Salmacis sphaeroides, 129, 131
Salmon sperm, 159
Sarcophyton elegans Moser, 83
Sarcophytum glaucum, 98, 99, 100, 101
Saxidomus giganteus, 75
Scymnus borealis, 73
Sepia officinalis, 169
Sinularia abrupta, 102
Sinularia flexibilis, 100
Sinularia gonatodes, 90
Solaster paxillatas, 72
Spatangus purpurens, 141
Spheciospongia vesparia, 63, 97
Spheroides rubripes, 163
Spongia nitens, 102, 103
Spongia officinalis obliqua, 99, 102, 103, 105, 149, 150
Stelleta clarella, 66, 68, 69, 73, 74, 75, 76, 78, 79, 80
Stichopus chloronotus Brandt, 113, 116
Stichopus japonicus Selenka, 111, 113, 115, 121, 124, 125, 126
Strombus gigas, 147
Strongylocentrotus sulcherrimus, 129
Stylatula sp., 109
Stylocheilus longicauda (Quoy and Gaimard), 141, 142
Suberites compacta, 72, 76
Sycon (or *Scypha*) *ciliatum*, 158, 160, 161
Tethya aurantia, 66, 69, 73, 74, 75, 76, 78, 79, 83
Tetrahymena pyriformis, 114, 146
Thelepus setosus, 87, 88, 127, 128, 134, 135, 154

Thelonota ananas Jaeger, 81, 82, 84, 85
Thorecta marginalis, 107, 108
Thorecta sp., 165
Thyone briareus, 150
Torpedo marmorata, 65
Tropiometra afra Hartlaub, 138
Turbo stenogyrus, 145
Verongia aurea Hyatt, 128
Verongia cauliformis, 128, 130
Verongia fistularis, 80, 128, 130
Verongia lacunosa, 164
Verongia sp., 130
Verongia spengelii, 165
Verongia thiona, 171, 172
Xiphigorgia anceps, 106
Xiphogergia sp., 80
Zoanthus confertus, 72
Zoanthus sociatus, 146

B. Marine Animal Components

Acanthasterol, 82
Acanthellin-1, 166
Acanthellin-2, 166
3-Acetamido-2,6-dibromo-3-hydroxy-2,6-cyclohexadiene-1-one, 128
3-Acetamido-2,6-dibromo-3-hydroxy -1,1-dimethoxycyclohexa-2,6-diene, 130
23-ξ-Acetoxy-17-deoxy-7,8-dihydroholothurino-genin, 116
Adenine, 153
Aequorin, 169
(+)-Aeroplysinin-1, 159
(−)-Aeroplysinin-1, 159
Aeroplysinin-2, 87
Aerothionin, 171
Africanol, 96
Agelasine, 172
Agmatine, 154
Alloxanthin, 118
2-Amino-3,4-dimethyl-6-dimethylamino-3H-1,3,5,7-tetraazacyclo-pent[f]azulene, 165

2-Amino-6-hydroxy-7,9-dimethylpurine betaine, 157

α-Amino-β-phosphono-propionic acid, 146

2-Aminoethanesulfonic acid, 145

3-(2-Aminoethyl)-5,6-dibromoindole, 161

2-Aminoethyl-phosphonic acid, 145

Amuresterol, 69

Anabaseine[2-(3-pyridyl)-3,4,5,6-tetra-hydropyridine], 161

Ancepsenolide, 106

Anhydroethylidene-3,3'-bis(2,6,7-trihydroxy-naphthazarin), 141

Anhydrofonsecin, 135

Anhydrofurospongin-1, 103

Anthopleurin A, 173

Aplysiatoxin, 141

Aplysin, 90

Aplysin-20, 102

Aplysinol, 90

Aplysinopsin, 165

Aplysterol, 80

1-β-D-Arabinofuranosyl-uracil, 160

1-β-D-Arabinosylthymine, 162

Arcaine, 156

Arcamine, 147

Arenicochrome, 19

9-Aristolene, 94

1(10)-Aristolene, 94

Asperdiol, 101

Astacin, 120

Astaxanthin, 121

Asterinsäure, 120

Asterosterol, 66

Avarol, 104

Avarone, 103

Axamide-1, 168

Axamide-2, 168

Axamide-4, 96

Axisonitrile-1, 167

Axisonitrile-2, 167

Axisonitrile-4, 96

Axisothiocyanate-1, 168

Axisothiocyanate-2, 168

Axisothiocyanate-4, 96

Biliverdin IX,α, 172

Bis-(3,5-dibromo-4-hydroxyphenyl)-methane, 134

Brassicasterol, 74

3-Bromo-5-chlorotyrosine, 148

6-Bromo-2-methyl-thioindoxyl sulfate, 159

4-Bromophakellin, 163

3-Bromotyrosine, 149

Callinecdysone A, 71

Callinecdysone B, 75

Calysterol, 77

Campesterol, 76

Cantharanthin, 121

$\Delta^{9(12)}$-Capnellene-3β,8β,10α-triol, 96

2-(13-Carboxy-14,15-diacetoxyhexadecanyl)-2-penten-4-olide, 109

α-Carotene, 122

β-Carotene, 122

γ-Carotene, 122

β-Carotene-4,4'-dione, 121

Cetyl palmitate, 63

5-Chlorocytosine, 152

5-Chlorodeoxycytidine, 159

3-Chlorotyrosine, 149

Cholestanol, 73

Cholesterol, 72

Choline, 155

Chondrillastanol, 74

Chondrillasterol, 78

Chondrillin, 107

ent-Chromazonarol, 104

Clionasterol, 80

Comantherin, 136

Comaparvin, 138

Comaparvin-3,6-disulfate ester, 138

Crassin acetate, 106

Crustecdysone, 71

Cynthiaxanthin, 118

Dactylene, 90

Dactyloxene B, 95

Debromoaplysiatoxin, 142

Debromorenierin-1, 62

Dehydrodendrolasin, 91

23-Demethyl-gorgosterol, 78

Dendrolasin, 92

6-Deoxy-D-glucose, 125

2-Deoxycrustecdysone, 71

17-Desoxy-12β-methoxy-7,8-dihydro-22,25-oxidoholothurinogenin-3-acetate, 117

17-Desoxy-22,25-oxidoholothurinogenin, 111

2,6-Dibromo-3-acetamidohydroquinone, 128

3,5-Dibromo-4-hydroxy-benzaldehyde, 127

3,5-Dibromo-4-hydroxy-benzyl alcohol, 128

4',6-Dibromo-2-hydroxy-diphenyl ether, 132

6,6'-Dibromo-indigotin, 166

Dibromophakellin, 162

2,6-Dibromophenol, 127

4,5-Dibromopyrrole-2-carboxylic acid, 147

3,5-Dibromotyrosine, 149

3,5-Dichlorotyrosine, 149

Dictyol A, 98

Dictyol B, 98

24,28-Didehydroaplysterol dps-1, 79

7,8-Didehydroastaxanthin, 120

Difurospinosulin, 114

Dihydrofurospongin-2, 103

Dihydronitenin, 103

18-Dihydrorenierin-1, 62

Dihydroxanthommatin, 169

2,7-Dihydroxy-6-acetyljuglone, 130

3,3'-Dihydroxy-ε-carotene, 123

2,6-Dihydroxy-3,7-dimethoxynaphthazarin, 133

2,7-Dihydroxy-3,6-dimethoxynaphthazarin, 133

2,7-Dihydroxy-3-ethylnaphthazarin, 133

2,5-Dihydroxy-3-ethylbenzoquinone, 128

(15S)-11,15-Dihydroxy-9-oxo-5-cis-13-trans-prostadienoic acid, 105

2,7-Dihydroxy-naphthazarin, 129

3,4-Dihydroxyquinoline-2-carboxylic acid, 160
3,5-Diiodotyrosine, 149
12β,25-Dimethoxy-7,8-dihydroholothurinogenin-3-acetate, 117
Dimethylamine, 151
4-Dimethylamino-1,2-dithiolane, 154
Dimethyl histamine, 157
1,3-Dimethyl-imidazole-4-acetic acid betaine, 157
1,3-Dimethylimidazole-4-carboxylic acid betaine, 155
Dimethyltaurine, 146
3,6-Dioxo-hexahydropyrrolo-[1,2-a]-pyrazine, 157
Dopamine, 158
α-Doradecin, 121
Dysidin, 166
Echinenone, 122
Echinochrome A, 134
Eledoisin, 173
(+)-β-Elemene, 94
Epinephrine, 160
Episterol, 74
Epizoanthoxanthin A, 164
Epizoanthoxanthin B, 165
Epoxynephthenol acetate, 106
Estradiol, 65
6-Ethyl-2,7-dihydroxy-2-methoxynaphthazarin, 134
Ethylamine, 151
Ethylidene-3,3′-bis(2,6,7-trihydroxynaphthazarin), 141
Eunicellin, 111
Eunicin, 99
Fasciculatin, 108
Flexibilene, 100
Fucoxanthinol, 123
Furospinosulin-1, 109
Furospinosulin-2, 112
Furospinosulin-3, 117
Furospongin-1, 105
Furospongin-2, 102
Furvoventalene, 89
(−)-Germacrene-A, 94
D-Glalactose, 125
D-Glucomethylose, 125

O-α-D-Glucopyranosyl-(1 → 2)-O-β-D-galactopyranosyloxy-(1 → 5)-L-lysine, 150
D-Glucose, 126
Glumethylose, 125
Glycocyamine, 145
Gorgastanone, 82
β-Gorgonene, 95
Gorgostane, 83
Gorgosterol, 82
Griseogenin, 113
Guanidine, 151
γ-Guanidino-butyric acid, 147
γ-Guanidino-β-hydroxybutyric acid, 148
Guanidoacetic acid, 145
β-Guanidinopropionic acid, 146
Gyrinal, 88
Hallachrome, 135
Heptacosane, 63
2-Heptapyrenyl-1,4-benzoquinone, 142
2-Heptapyrenyl-1,4-quinol, 143
Herbipoline, 157
Hercynine, 160
Heteronemin, 77
Hexadecanol, 62
2-Hexapyrenyl-1,4-benzoquinone, 142
2-Hexapyrenyl-1,4-quinol, 118
Histamine, 153
Histidine, 148
Holothurinogenin, 112
Holotoxin A, 124
Holotoxinogenin, 113
Holotoxinogenin 25-methyl ether, 115
Homoaerothionin, 172
Homarine, 156
2-Hydroxy-3-acetyl-7-methoxynaphthazarin, 134
2-Hydroxy-3-acetylnaphthazarin, 131
12α-Hydroxy-7,8-dihydro-24,25-dehydroholothurinogenin, 111
2-Hydroxy-6-ethyljuglone, 132

2-Hydroxy-3-ethylnaphthazarin, 132
2-Hydroxy-6-ethylnaphthazarin, 132
(15R)-15-Hydroxy-9-oxo-5-*cis*-10,13-*trans*-prostatrienoic acid, 99
(15S)-15-Hydroxy-9-oxo-5-*cis*-10,13-*trans*-prostatrienoic acid, 100
(15S)-15-Hydroxy-9-oxo-5-*trans*-10,13-*trans*-prostatrienoic acid, 100
9-Hydroxy-3-tetrapyrenylbenzoic acid, 110
Hydroxyancepsenolide, 106
γ-Hydroxyarginine, 156
24-Hydroxyircinolide, 108
25-Hydroxymethyl-2-octapyrenyl-1,4-quinol, 143
2-Hydroxynephthenol, 101
4-Hydroxyphenyl-pyruvic acid oxime, 159
18-Hydroxyrenierin-2, 63
5-Hydroxytryptamine, 161
Icrinolide, 107
Imidazolyl acrylic acid, 155
Imidazolyl lactic acid, 156
Inositol, 126
3-Iodotyrosine, 150
Ircinin-1, 108
Ircinin-2, 108
Ircinin-3, 104
Ircinin-4, 104
Isoagatholactone, 99
Isoamylamine, 154
Isochodoptilometrin, 137
3-Isocyano-3,7,11,15-tetramethyl-1,6,10,14-hexadecatetraene, 170
9-Isocyanopupukeanane, 167
Isodactylyne, 91
Isofurospongin-2, 103
6-Isopropyl-3,9,13-trimethylcyclotetradec-2,7,9,12-tetraene-1-ol, 100
6-Isopropyl-3,9,13-trimethylcyclotetradec-2,7,12-triene-1,9-diol, 101
Isorenieratene, 119

3-Isothiocyano-3,7,11,15-
tetramethyl-1,6,10,14-
hexadecatetraene, 170
Kitol, 123
Koellikerigenin, 113
Lathosterol, 72
Lobolide, 105
Lobophytolide, 97
Longifolin, 90
Luciferin, 170
Lutein, 119
Lysine, 148
(+)-γ-Maaliene, 95
Metanethole, 97
5-Methoxy-comaparvin,
139
5-Methoxy-comaparvin-
3,6-disulfate ester, 139
5-Methoxycomaparvin-6-
methyl ether, 140
5-Methoxycomaparvin-6-
methyl ether 3-sulfate
ester, 140
25-Methoxy-17-
desoxyholothurinogenin,
115
12α-Methoxy-7,8-dihydro-
17-desoxy-22,25-
oxidoholothurinogenin,
115
12β-Methoxy-7,8-dihydro-
24,25-dehydro-
holothurinogenin-3-
acetate, 118
12β-Methoxy-7,8-dihydro-
22-hydroxyholo-
thurinogenin, 116
12β-Methoxy-7,8-dihydro-
22,25-oxido-
holothurinogenin, 116
12β-Methoxy-7,8-
dihydroholothurinogenin-
3,22-diacetate, 117
3-Methoxy-D-glucose, 126
25-Methoxyholothurino-
genin, 116
1-Methyl-adenine, 155
Methyl (15R)-15-
Hydroxy-5-*cis*-10,13-
trans-prostatrienoate
15-acetate, 107
2-Methyl-8-hydroxy-2H-
pyrano(3,2-g)-
naphthazarin, 135

N-Methyl-nicotinic acid,
157
N-Methyl-picolinic acid,
156
Methyl *trans*-
monocyclofarnesate, 97
2-*N*-Methylamino-3-
(ethyl)-indole, 163
2-Methylamino-
ethylphosphonic acid,
146
24-Methylenecholest-5-en-
3β,7β,19-triol, 76
3-O-Methylglucose, 126
Microcionin-1, 92
Microcionin-2, 93
Microcionin-3, 93
Microcionin-4, 93
Monomethyltaurine, 146
Murexine, 164
Namakochrome, 130
Naphthopurpurin, 128
Navenone A, 166
Navenone B, 61
Navenone C, 61
Neocemantherin, 138
Neospongosterol, 76
Nephthenol, 101
Nereistoxin, 154
Nitenin, 102
Norepinephrine, 158
3-Norpseudo-
zoanthoxanthin, 163
Norzooanemonin, 155
Octadecanol, 62
2-Octapyrenyl-1,4-
benzoquinone, 143
2-Octapyrenyl-1,4-quinol,
143
Octopamine, 158
Octopine, 160
Oroidin, 162
22,25-Oxido-
holothurinogenin, 112
Oxyluciferin, 169
Pachydictyol A, 101
Pahutoxin, 171
Pallescensin-1, 93
Pallescensin-2, 91
Pallescensin-3, 92
Pallescensin A, 93
Pallescensin B, 91
Pallescensin C, 89
Pallescensin D, 89

Pallescensin E, 88
Pallescensin F, 89
Pallescensin G, 89
Paracentione, 114
Paragracine, 165
Parazoanthoxanthin A, 161
Parazoanthoxanthin D, 164
Pectenolone, 121
Pectenoxanthin, 118
1,2,3,1',3'-Pentabromo-5-
hydroxyphenyl ether,
130
Peridinin, 119
Pleraplysillin, 92
Pleraplysillin-2, 97
Poriferastanol, 74
Praslinogenin, 116
Prepacifenol, 92
Pristane, 97
3-Propionyl-1,6,8-
trihydroxy-9,10-
anthraquinone, 136
3-Propyl-1,6,8-
trihydroxy-9,10-
anthraquinone, 136
Propylamine, 151
Provitamine A, 123
Pseudozoanthoxanthin, 164
Ptilometric acid, 138
Ptilosarcenone, 107
Ptilosarcone, 110
Pukalide, 102
Putrescine, 152
D-Quinovose, 125
Renieratene, 120
Renierin-1, 62
Renierin-2, 63
Rhodocomatulin 6,8-
dimethyl ether, 140
Rhodocomatulin 6-
monomethyl ether, 139
Rhodoptilometrin, 137
Rubrocomatulin
monomethyl ether, 139
Sarcophine, 98
Saxitoxin, 162
Scalaradiol, 110
Scalarin, 110
Scymanol, 73
(−)-β-Selinene, 95
Serotonin, 161
Seychellogenin, 112
Sinulariolide, 100
β-Sitosterol, 80

Sodium comantheryl
  sulfate, 136
Spiniferin-1, 88
Spiniferin-2, 88
Spinochrome A, 131
Spinochrome B, 129
Spinochrome C, 132
Spinochrome D, 129
Spinochrome E, 129
Spinochrome G, 131
Spinochrome S, 131
Spongopurine, 155
Spongosine, 163
Spongothymidine, 162
Spongouridine, 160
trans-Squalene, 114
Stellasterol, 75
Stichopogenin A_2, 111
Stichopogenin A_4, 113
Strombine, 147
Stylatulide, 109
Surugatoxin, 171
Taurine, 145
Taurobetaine, 148
Taurocyamine, 146
Ternaygenin, 115
Tetradecanol, 61
7,7',8,8'-Tetradehydro-
  astaxanthin, 120
Tetrahydrofurospongin-2,
  105
Tetrahymanol, 114
3,7,11,15-Tetramethyl-
  1,6,10,14-hexadeca-
  tetraene-3-formamide,
  170
Tetramine, 152
2-Tetraprenyl-1,4-
  benzoquinone, 110
Tetrodotoxin, 163
Thelephenol, 88
Thelepin, 87
Thornasterol A, 71
Thornasterol B, 76
Thymine, 153
2,4,6-Tribromophenol,
  127
Trigonelline, 157
2,3,7-Trihydroxy-6-
  acetyljuglone, 131
2,3,7-Trihydroxy-6-
  ethyljuglone, 133
2,6,7-Trihydroxy-3-
  ethyljuglone, 133

S(−)-1,6,8-Trihydroxy-3-
  (1-hydroxypropyl)-
  anthraquinone, 137
3β,20ξ,25-Trihydroxy-16-
  oxolanost-9(11)-ene-18-
  carboxylic acid lactone
  (18 → 20), 113
Trimethylamine, 152
2-Trimethylaminoethyl-
  phosphonic acid betaine,
  154
Tyramine, 158
Tyrosine, 150
Uracil, 152
Urocanic acid, 155
Urocanylcholine, 164
Variabilin, 109
Xanthommatin, 169
Xanthophyll, 119
D-Xylose, 125
3β-Xyloside-12β-methoxy-
  7,8-dihydro-24,25-
  dehydroholothurino-
  genin, 118
Zeaxanthin, 119
Zoanthoxanthin, 165
Zooanemonine, 157

Molecular Weights

A. PLANTS

162, 21
182, 21
184, 35
194, 35
224, 35
232, 9
256, 22
262, 9
266, 23
270, 21, 22
301, 36
314, 10, 22
315, 36
328, 23
330, 9, 10, 22
344, 23
346, 10
348, 11, 24, 27
352, 23
358, 24
360, 10
362, 24, 25

364, 11
374, 24
378, 19, 27
384, 19
392, 36
394, 11
436, 12
442, 11, 12, 13
456, 13
468, 25
473, 37
478, 12
484, 20
493, 37
528, 37, 38
530, 38
536, 12
562, 13, 28
576, 28
590, 14
592, 28
594, 28, 29
606, 29
608, 29, 30
610, 30
622, 31
624, 31
638, 31
648, 14
652, 14, 33
680, 17
683, 30
774, 15
787, 39
800, 36
804, 14
886, 15
890, 15
892, 32
904, 32
1012, 15

B. MARINE ANIMALS

45, 151
59, 151, 152
87, 154
88, 152
91, 152
101, 154
111, 153
112, 152
117, 145, 147
121, 155
125, 145

126, 153
130, 154
131, 146
135, 153
137, 156, 157, 158
138, 155
139, 146, 157
140, 155, 156
145, 147, 152
146, 148
147, 147
149, 154, 155
150, 125
153, 146, 158
154, 157
155, 148
156, 156
160, 161
161, 148, 158
164, 125
167, 146, 148, 154
168, 128
169, 146, 158
172, 156
176, 161
179, 157
180, 125, 126
181, 150
183, 160
190, 156
194, 126
195, 159
196, 41
197, 160
204, 94, 95
205, 160
206, 128
210, 147
212, 88
214, 61, 89, 161
215, 149
216, 91, 92
218, 92, 93, 132
222, 96, 129
224, 61
225, 166
228, 163
229, 96
230, 90
231, 166, 167
234, 88, 132
236, 95
238, 129
240, 61

241, 164
242, 62, 164
244, 160
246, 90, 160
247, 96
248, 92, 130, 131
249, 168, 169
250, 97, 133, 149, 152
252, 96, 127
254, 41, 129, 165
256, 164, 165
258, 162
260, 149
261, 96, 159
263, 168
264, 131
268, 97, 130, 134, 135, 153
269, 147
270, 62, 165
272, 65, 100, 135
274, 135
277, 169
278, 134
280, 127, 132, 134
282, 41, 128, 133
283, 155, 162
286, 136
288, 100, 101
290, 101
295, 90, 148
296, 97
297, 163
298, 136
299, 170
300, 138
302, 98, 99
306, 101
307, 150
310, 163
311, 90
312, 103, 136
314, 62, 104, 137, 138
316, 97, 98
317, 170
318, 161
319, 163
320, 101
325, 128
326, 102, 103
328, 97, 103
330, 63, 105, 139
331, 127, 170
332, 65, 163
334, 99, 100

338, 159
339, 149, 159
340, 87, 102
342, 103, 138, 140
344, 104, 132, 140
346, 63
348, 106
354, 66, 109
356, 139
360, 141
362, 106
366, 105
368, 66
370, 43, 66, 67, 140
371, 130
372, 67, 102, 139
374, 105
376, 106
380, 63, 106, 107
382, 68, 107
384, 69
385, 130
386, 72
387, 102
388, 73, 136
389, 162
394, 62, 169
396, 62, 73, 74, 110
397, 166
398, 68, 74, 75, 108, 109
400, 76, 77
402, 77
405, 170
408, 108
410, 77, 78, 108, 110, 114
411, 90
412, 65, 78, 79, 83, 91, 107
414, 68, 75, 80
416, 70, 77, 81
418, 72
420, 166
422, 112
424, 140
426, 82, 83
428, 67, 74, 79, 110, 114
430, 76
432, 71
433, 149
436, 73, 171
440, 81
443, 169
444, 110
445, 92, 169
446, 76

448, 114
450, 73
452, 164
454, 112
458, 172
460, 138
462, 114
464, 71
465, 87
467, 88, 135
468, 111
470, 81, 112, 113
472, 81
478, 87
480, 63, 71, 107
482, 109
484, 111, 112, 115, 141
486, 113, 150
488, 77, 82, 83
490, 117, 139
492, 83
494, 75
500, 115, 116

502, 141
508, 83
512, 84
514, 84, 116
516, 116, 134, 142
518, 116, 118
522, 111
528, 119, 120
530, 85
536, 118, 119, 122
540, 119
542, 109, 117
550, 122
551, 85
564, 121
568, 110, 123
572, 123
574, 117
578, 117
580, 121
581, 130
584, 142, 172
586, 143

590, 118
592, 120, 142
594, 120
596, 121
616, 123
630, 119
634, 142
649, 118
652, 143
654, 143
670, 143
671, 141
684, 171
713, 142
818, 171
832, 172
929, 172
1064, 85
1187, 173
1318, 124
5086, 173
22,000–24,000, 173

Bibliography

1. D. Ackermann and C. Burchard. *Hoppe-Seylers Z. Physiol. Chem.* **271**, 183 (1941).
2. D. Ackermann, F. Holtz, and H. Reinwein. *Z. Biol.* **82**, 278 (1924) [*Chem. Abstr.* **19**, 2090 (1925)].
3. D. Ackermann, F. Holtz, and H. Reinwein. *Z. Biol.* **79**, 113 (1923) [*Chem. Abstr.* **18**, 1133 (1924)].
4. D. Ackermann and P. H. List, *Naturwissenschaften* **48**, 74 (1961).
5. D. Ackermann and P. H. List. *Naturwissenschaften* **46**, 354 (1959).
6. D. Ackermann and P. H. List. *Naturwissenschaften* **44**, 513 (1957).
7. D. Ackermann and P. H. List. *Naturwissenschaften* **44**, 184 (1957).
8. D. Ackermann and P. H. List. *Hoppe-Seylers Z. Physiol. Chem.* **323**, 192 (1961).
9. D. Ackermann and P. H. List. *Hoppe-Seylers Z. Physiol. Chem.* **318**, 281 (1960).
10. D. Ackermann and P. H. List. *Hoppe-Seylers Z. Physiol. Chem.* **317**, 78 (1959).
11. D. Ackermann and P. H. List. *Hoppe-Seylers Z. Physiol. Chem.* **309**, 286 (1957).
12. D. Ackermann and P. H. List. *Hoppe-Seylers Z. Physiol. Chem.* **308**, 270 (1957).
13. D. Ackermann, P. H. List, and H. G. Menssen. *Hoppe-Seylers Z. Physiol. Chem.* **312**, 210 (1958).
14. D. Ackermann and H. G. Menssen. *Hoppe-Seylers Z. Physiol. Chem.* **322**, 198 (1960).
15. D. Ackermann and E. Müller. *Hoppe-Seylers Z. Physiol. Chem.* **269**, 146 (1941).
16. D. Ackermann and R. Pant. *Hoppe-Seylers Z. Physiol. Chem.* **326**, 197 (1961).
17. M. Adinolfi, L. De Napoli, B. Di Blasio, A. Iengo, C. Pedone, and C. Santacroce. *Tetrahedron Lett.* 2815 (1977).
18. S. Akasi. *J. Biochem. Tokyo* **25**, 261 (1937).
19. A. Anastasi and V. Erspamer. *Arch. Biochem. Biophys.* **101**, 56 (1963).
20. R. J. Andersen and D. J. Faulkner. *Tetrahedron Lett.* 1175 (1973).
21. H. A. Anderson, J. Smith, and R. H. Thomson. *J. Chem. Soc.* 2141 (1965).
22. M. M. Anisimov, E. B. Fronert, T. A. Kuzunetsova, and G. B. Elyakov, *Toxicon* **11**, 109 (1973).
23. F. Arcamone. *Lloydia* **40**, 45 (1977).
24. R. B. Ashworth and M. J. Cormier. *Science* **155**, 1558 (1967).
25. J. Avigan and M. Blumer. *J. Lipid Res.* **9**, 350 (1968).
26. J. T. Baker and V. Murphy. Volume 1, "Compounds from Marine Organisms, Section II. Marine Products" in *CRC Handbook of Marine Science*, CRC Press, 1976.
27. J. T. Baker and M. D. Sutherland. *Tetrahedron Lett.* 43 (1968).
28. J. A. Ballantine, J. C. Roberts, and R. J. Morris. *Tetrahedron Lett.* 105 (1975).
29. J. A. Ballantine, K. Williams, and B. A. Burke. *Tetrahedron Lett.* 1547 (1977).
30. G. L. Bartolini, T. R. Erdman, and P. J. Scheuer. *Tetrahedron* **29**, 3699 (1973).
31. D. Becher, C. Djerassi, R. E. Moore, H. Singh, and P. J. Scheuer. *J. Org. Chem.* **31**, 3650 (1966).

32. C. M. Beechan and C. Djerassi. *Tetrahedron Lett.* 2395 (1977).
33. M. A. Beno, R. H. Cox, J. M. Wells, R. J. Cole, J. W. Kirksey, and G. G. Christoph. *J. Amer. Chem. Soc.* **99**, 4123 (1977).
34. L. Béress, R. Béress, and G. Wunderer. *Toxicon* **13**, 359 (1975).
35. W. Bergmann and D. C. Burke. *J. Org. Chem.* **21**, 226 (1956).
36. W. Bergmann and D. C. Burke. *J. Org. Chem.* **20**, 1501 (1955).
37. W. Bergmann and R. J. Feeney. *J. Amer. Chem. Soc.* **72**, 2809 (1950).
38. W. Bergmann and R. J. Feeney. *J. Org. Chem.* **16**, 981 (1951).
39. W. Bergmann, R. J. Feeney, and A. N. Swift. *J. Org. Chem.* **16**, 1337 (1951).
40. W. Bergmann, D. H. Gould, and E. M. Low, *J. Org. Chem.* **10**, 570 (1945).
41. W. Bergmann and W. J. McAleer, *J. Amer. Chem. Soc.* **73**, 4969 (1951).
42. W. Bergmann, M. J. McLean, and D. Lester. *J. Org. Chem.* **8**, 271 (1963).
43. W. Bergmann and F. H. McTigue. *J. Org. Chem.* **13**, 738 (1948).
44. W. Bergmann and W. T. Pace. *J. Amer. Chem. Soc.* **65**, 477 (1943).
45. W. Bergmann and M. F. Stempien, Jr. *J. Org. Chem.* **22**, 1575 (1957).
46. J. Bernstein, U. Shmeuli, E. Zadock, Y. Kashman, and I. Neeman. *Tetrahedron* **30**, 2817 (1974).
47. J. H. Block. *Steroids* **23**, 421 (1974).
48. A. Bolognese and G. Scherillo. *Experientia* **30**, 225 (1974).
49. D. B. Borders, G. O. Morton, and E. R. Wetzel. *Tetrahedron Lett.* 2709 (1974).
50. M. Bortolotto, J. C. Braekman, D. Daloze, D. Losman, and B. Tursch. *Steroids* **28**, 461 (1976).
51. D. B. Boylan and P. J. Scheuer. *Science* **155**, 52 (1967).
52. J. C. Braekman, D. Daloze, R. Ottinger, and B. Tursch. *Experientia* **33**, 993 (1977).
53. H. Bredereck, O. Christmann, and W. Koser. *Chem. Ber.* **93**, 1206 (1960).
54. J. Breuer and H. Breuer. *Naturwissenschaften* **55**, 391 (1968).
55. D. M. Brown, A. Todd, and S. Varadarajan. *J. Chem. Soc.* **2388** (1956).
56. G. L. Bundy, E. G. Daniels, F. H. Lincoln, and J. E. Pike, *J. Amer. Chem. Soc.* **94**, 2124 (1972).
57. B. J. Burreson, C. Christophersen, and P. J. Scheuer. *J. Amer. Chem. Soc.* **97**, 201 (1975).
58. B. J. Burreson, C. Christophersen, and P. J. Scheuer. *Tetrahedron* **31**, 2015 (1975).
59. B. J. Burreson and P. J. Scheuer. *J.C.S. Chem. Commun.* 1035 (1974).
60. B. J. Burreson, P. J. Scheuer, J. Finer, and J. Clardy. *J. Amer. Chem. Soc.* **97**, 4763 (1975).
61. A. Butenandt, U. Schiedt, and E. Biekert. *Justus Liebigs Ann. Chem.* **588**, 106 (1954).
62. F. Cafieri, L. De Napoli, E. Fattorusso, and C. Santacroce. *Experientia* **33**, 994 (1977).
63. F. Cafieri, L. De Napoli, E. Fattorusso, C. Santacroce, and D. Sica. *Gazz. Chim. Ital.* **107**, 71 (1977).
64. F. Cafieri, E. Fattorusso, A. Frigerio, C. Santacroce, and D. Sica. *Gazz. Chim. Ital.* **105**, 595 (1975).
65. F. Cafieri, E. Fattorusso, S. Magno, C. Santacroce, and D. Sica. *Tetrahedron* **29**, 4259 (1973).
66. F. Cafieri, E. Fattorusso, C. Santacroce, and L. Minale. *Tetrahedron* **28**, 1579 (1972).
67. S. A. Campbell, A. K. Mallams, E. S. Waight, B. C. L. Weedon, M. Barbier, E. Lederer, and A. Salaque. *J.C.S. Chem. Commun.* 941 (1967).
68. L. Cariello, S. Crescenzi, G. Prota, S. Capasso, F. Giordano, and L. Mazzarella. *Tetrahedron* **30**, 3281 (1974).
69. L. Cariello, S. Crescenzi, G. Prota, F. Giordano, and L. Mazzarella. *J.C.S. Chem. Commun.* 99 (1973).

70. L. Cariello, S. Crescenzi, G. Prota, and L. Zanetti. *Experientia* **30**, 849 (1974).
71. L. Cariello, S. Crescenzi, G. Prota, and L. Zanetti. *Tetrahedron* **30**, 4191 (1974).
72. S. K. Carter and R. B. Livingston. *Cancer Treatment Reports* **60**, 1141 (1976).
73. J. M. Cassady and H. G. Floss. *Lloydia* **40**, 90 (1977).
74. C. W. J. Chang, R. E. Moore, and P. J. Scheuer. *J. Amer. Chem. Soc.* **86**, 2959 (1964).
75. C. W. J. Chang, R. E. Moore, and P. J. Scheuer. *Tetrahedron Lett.* 3557 (1964).
76. J. D. Chanley, R. Ledeen, J. Wax, R. F. Nigrelli, and H. Sobotka. *J. Amer. Chem. Soc.* **81**, 5180 (1959).
77. J. D. Chanley, T. Mezzetti, and H. Sobotka. *Tetrahedron* **22**, 1857 (1966).
78. J. D. Chanley and C. Rossi. *Tetrahedron* **25**, 1911 (1969).
79. J. D. Chanley and C. Rossi. *Tetrahedron* **25**, 1897 (1969).
80. L. T. Ch'ien, F. M. Shabel, Jr., and C. A. Alford, Jr. "Arabinosyl Nucleosides and Nucleotides," in *Selective Inhibitors of Viral Functions*, CRC Press, 1975, p. 227.
81. L. S. Ciereszko, M. A. Johnson, R. W. Schmidt, and C. B. Koons. *Comp. Biochem. Physiol.* **24**, 899 (1968).
82. G. Cimino, D. De Rosa, S. De Stefano, and L. Minale. *Tetrahedron* **30**, 645 (1974).
83. G. Cimino and S. De Stefano. *Tetrahedron Lett.* 1325 (1977).
84. G. Cimino, S. De Stefano, A. Guerriero, and L. Minale. *Tetrahedron Lett.* 3723 (1975).
85. G. Cimino, S. De Stefano, A. Guerriero, L. Minale. *Tetrahedron Lett.* 1425 (1975).
86. G. Cimino, S. De Stefano, A. Guerriero, and L. Minale. *Tetrahedron Lett.* 1421 (1975).
87. G. Cimino, S. De Stefano, A. Guerriero, and L. Minale. *Tetrahedron Lett.* 1417 (1975).
88. G. Cimino, S. De Stefano, and L. Minale. *Experientia* **31**, 1117 (1975).
89. G. Cimino, S. De Stefano, and L. Minale. *Experientia* **31**, 756 (1975).
90. G. Cimino, S. De Stefano, and L. Minale. *Experientia* **30**, 846 (1974).
91. G. Cimino, S. De Stefano, and L. Minale. *Experientia* **29**, 1063 (1973).
92. G. Cimino, S. De Stefano, and L. Minale. *Experientia* **28**, 1401 (1972).
93. G. Cimino, S. De Stefano, and L. Minale. *Tetrahedron* **28**, 5983 (1972).
94. G. Cimino, S. De Stefano, and L. Minale. *Tetrahedron* **28**, 1315 (1972).
95. G. Cimino, S. De Stefano, L. Minale, and E. Fattorusso. *Tetrahedron* **28**, 333 (1972)
96. G. Cimino, S. De Stefano, L. Minale, and E. Fattorusso. *Tetrahedron* **28**, 267 (1972).
97. G. Cimino, S. De Stefano, L. Minale, and E. Fattorusso. *Tetrahedron* **27**, 4673 (1971).
98. G. Cimino, S. De Stefano, L. Minale, and E. Trivellone. *Tetrahedron Lett.* 3727 (1975).
99. G. Cimino, S. De Stefano, L. Minale, and E. Trivellone. *Tetrahedron* **28**, 4761 (1972).
100. J. R. Cole, S. J. Torrance, R. M. Wiedhopf, S. K. Arora, and R. B. Bates. *J. Org. Chem.* **41**, 1852 (1976).
101. J. C. Coll, G. B. Hawes, N. Liyanage, W. Oberhänsli, and R. J. Wells. *Aust. J. Chem.* **30**, 1305 (1977).
102. J. C. Coll, S. J. Mitchell, and G. J. Stokie. *Tetrahedron Lett.* 1539 (1977).
103. G. A. Cordell, P. T. O. Chang, H. H. S. Fong, and N. R. Farnsworth. *Lloydia* **40**, 340 (1977).
104. G. A. Cordell and N. R. Farnsworth. *Lloydia* **40**, 1 (1977).
105. G. A. Cordell and N. R. Farnsworth. *Heterocycles* **4**, 393 (1976).
106. D. B. Cosulich and F. M. Lovell. *J.C.S. Chem. Commun.* 397 (1971).

107. H. D. Crone, B. Leake, M. W. Jarvis, and S. E. Freeman. *Toxicon* **14**, 423 (1976).
108. A. D. Cross. *J. Chem. Soc.* 2817 (1961).
109. E. Cullen and J. P. Devlin. *Can. J. Chem.* **53**, 1690 (1975).
110. P. De Luca, M. De Rosa, L. Minale, and G. Sodano. *J.C.S. Perkin Trans I* 2132 (1972).
111. S. De Rosa, L. Minale, R. Riccio, and G. Sodano. *J.C.S. Perkin Trans I* 1408 (1976).
112. C. Djerassi, R. M. K. Carlson, S. Popov, and T. H. Varkony. "Sterols from Marine Sources" in *Marine Natural Products Chemistry*, Ed. by D. J. Faulkner and W. H. Fenical, Plenum Publishing Corp., New York, N.Y., 1977, p. 111.
113. J. D. Douros. *Cancer Treatment Reports* **60**, 1069 (1976).
114. P. J. Drum, W. F. O'Connor, and L. P. Renouf. *Biochem. J.* **39**, 208 (1945).
115. G. B. Elyakov, T. A. Kuznetsova, A. K. Dzizenko, and Yu. N. Elkin. *Tetrahedron Lett.* 1151 (1969).
116. G. B. Elyakov, T. A. Kuznetsova, and V. E. Vaskovskii. *Chem. Natur. Compds. USSR* **4**, 253 (1968).
117. J. P. Engelbrecht, B. Tursch, and C. Djerassi. *Steroids* **20**, 121 (1972).
118. E. L. Enwall, D. Van Der Helm, I. N. Hsu, T. Pattabhiraman, F. J. Schmitz, R. L. Spraggins, and A. J. Weinheimer. *J.C.S. Chem. Commun.* 215 (1972).
119. T. R. Erdman and R. H. Thomson. *Tetrahedron* **28**, 5163 (1972).
120. V. Erspamer and A. Anastasi. *Experientia* **18**, 58 (1962).
121. V. Erspamer and O. Benati. *Science* **117**, 161 (1953).
122. V. Erspamer and G. Boretti. *Arch. Int. Pharmacodyn. Ther.* **87**, 296 (1951) [*Chem. Abstr.* **46**, 2700h (1952)].
123. U. H. M. Fagerlund and D. R. Idler. *J. Amer. Chem. Soc.* **81**, 401 (1959).
124. U. H. M. Fagerlund and D. R. Idler. *J. Amer. Chem. Soc.* **79**, 6473 (1957).
125. U. H. M. Fagerlund and D. R. Idler. *J. Org. Chem.* **21**, 372 (1956).
126. E. Fattorusso, S. Forenza, L. Minale, and G. Sodano. *Gazz. Chim. Ital.* **101**, 104 (1971).
127. E. Fattorusso, S. Magno, L. Mayol, C. Santacroce, and D. Sica. *Tetrahedron* **31**, 1715 (1975).
128. E. Fattorusso, S. Magno, L. Mayol, C. Santacroce, and D. Sica. *Tetrahedron* **31**, 269 (1975).
129. E. Fattorusso, S. Magno, L. Mayol, C. Santacroce, and D. Sica. *Tetrahedron* **30**, 3911 (1974).
130. E. Fattorusso, S. Magno, C. Santacroce, and D. Sica. *Gazz. Chim. Ital.* **104**, 409 (1974).
131. E. Fattorusso, S. Magno, C. Santacroce, and D. Sica. *Tetrahedron* **28**, 5993 (1972).
132. E. Fattorusso, L. Minale, K. Moody, G. Sodano, and R. H. Thomson. *Gazz. Chim. Ital.* **101**, 61 (1971).
133. E. Fattorusso, L. Minale, and G. Sodano. *J.C.S. Perkin Trans* 1 16 (1972).
134. E. Fattorusso, L. Minale, and G. Sodano. *J.C.S. Chem. Commun.* 751 (1970).
135. E. Fattorusso, L. Minale, G. Sodano, K. Moody, and R. H. Thomson. *J.C.S. Chem. Commun.* 752 (1970).
136. E. Fattorusso, L. Minale, G. Sodano, and E. Trivellone. *Tetrahedron* **27**, 3909 (1971).
137. D. J. Faulkner. *Tetrahedron* **33**, 1421 (1977).
138. D. J. Faulkner. *Pure Appl. Chem.* **48**, 25 (1976).
139. D. J. Faulkner. *Tetrahedron Lett.* 3821 (1973).
140. D. J. Faulkner and W. H. Fenical. *Marine Natural Products Chemistry*, NATO Conference Series IV: Marine Sciences Press, New York, 1977.
141. D. J. Faulkner, M. O. Stallard, J. Fayos, and J. Clardy. *J. Amer. Chem. Soc.* **95** 3413 (1973).
142. D. J. Faulkner, M. O. Stallard, and C. Ireland. *Tetrahedron Lett.* 3571 (1974).

143. A. Faux, D. H. S. Horn, E. J. Middleton, H. M. Fales, and M. E. Lowe. *J.C.S. Chem. Commun.* 175 (1969).
144. E. Fernholz and W. L. Ruigh. *J. Amer. Chem. Soc.* **63**, 1157 (1941).
145. E. Fernholz and W. L. Ruigh. *J. Amer. Chem. Soc.* **62**, 3346 (1940).
146. P. Fernlund and L. Josefsson. *Science* **177**, 173 (1972).
147. S. Forenza, L. Minale, R. Riccio, and E. Fattorusso. *J.C.S. Chem. Commun.* 1129 (1971).
148. G. W. Francis, R. R. Upadhyay, and S. Liaaen-Jensen. *Acta Chem. Scand.* **24**, 3050 (1970).
149. M. Fryberg, A. C. Oehlschlager, and A. M. Unrau. *J.C.S. Chem. Commun.* 204 (1972).
150. M. Fryberg, A. C. Oehlschlager, and A. M. Unrau. *J.C.S. Chem. Commun.* 1194 (1971).
151. E. Fujita, Y. Nagao, K. Kaneko, S. Nakazawa, and H. Kuroda. *Chem. Pharm. Bull. Tokyo* **24**, 2118 (1976).
152. Y. Fukuyama, C. L. Kirkemo, and J. D. White. *J. Amer. Chem. Soc.* **99**, 646 (1977).
153. W. Fulmer, G. E. Van Lear, G. O. Morton, and R. D. Mills. *Tetrahedron Lett.* 4551 (1970).
154. J. Fuska. *J. Antibiot. Tokyo* **22**, 365 (1977).
155. G. Galasko, J. Hora, T. P. Toube, B. C. L. Weedon, D. Andre, M. Barbier, E. Lederer, and V. R. Villanueva. *J. Chem. Soc. (C)*, 1264 (1969).
156. M. N. Galbraith, D. H. S. Horn, E. J. Middleton, and R. J. Hackney. *J.C.S. Chem. Commun.* 466 (1968).
157. M. N. Galbraith, D. H. S. Horn, E. J. Middleton, and R. J. Hackney. *J.C.S. Chem. Commun.* 83 (1968).
158. E. L. Gasteiger, P. C. Haake, and J. A. Gergen. *Ann. N.Y. Acad. Sci.* **90**, 622 (1960).
159. P. C. Ghosh, J. E. Larrahondo, P. W. LeQuesne, and R. F. Raffauf. *Lloydia* **40**, 364 (1977).
160. C. Giannotti, B. C. Das, and E. Lederer. *Bull. Soc. Chim. Fr.* **9**, 3299 (1966).
161. T. Goto, Y. Kishi, S. Takahashi, and Y. Hirata. *Tetrahedron* **21**, 2059 (1965).
162. J. H. Gough and M. D. Sutherland. *Aust. J. Chem.* **23**, 1839 (1970).
163. J. H. Gough and M. D. Sutherland. *Aust. J. Chem.* **20**, 1693 (1967).
164. J. H. Gough and M. D. Sutherland. *Tetrahedron Lett.* 269 (1964).
165. P. T. Grant and A. M. Mackie. *Nature* **267**, 786 (1977).
166. J. S. Grossert, P. Mathiaparanam, G. D. Hebb, P. Price, and I. M. Campbell. *Experientia* **29**, 258 (1973).
167. K. C. Gupta and P. J. Scheuer. *Steroids* **13**, 343 (1969).
168. K. C. Gupta and P. J. Scheuer. *Tetrahedron* **24**, 5831 (1968).
169. G. Habermehl and G. Volkwein. *Justus Liebigs An. Chem.* **731**, 53 (1970).
170. G. Habermehl and C. Volkwein. *Naturwissenschaften* **55**, 83 (1968).
171. R. L. Hale, J. Leclercq, B. Tursch, C. Djerassi, R. A. Gross, Jr., A. J. Weinheimer, K. Gupta, and P. J. Scheuer. *J. Amer. Chem. Soc.* **92**, 2179 (1970).
172. F. Hampshire and D. H. S. Horn. *J.C.S. Chem. Commun.* 37 (1966).
173. L. J. Haňka and A. Dietz. *J. Antibot. Tokyo* **29**, 611 (1976).
174. W. J. Hartman, W. G. Clark, S. D. Cyr, A. L. Jordon, and R. A. Leibhold. *Ann. N.Y. Acad. Sci.* **90**, 637 (1960).
175. J. L. Hartwell. *Cancer Treatment Reports* **60**, 1031 (1976).
176. T. H. Haskell. *Ann. N.Y. Acad. Sci.* **284**, 81 (1977).
177. Y. Hayashi, Y. Yūki, T. Matsumoto, and T. Sakan. *Tetrahedron Lett.* 2953 (1977).
178. M. Hérin, M. Colin, and B. Tursch. *Bull. Soc. Chim. Belg.* **85**, 801 (1976).
179. T. Higa and P. J. Scheuer. *Tetrahedron* **31**, 2379 (1975).
180. T. Higa and P. J. Scheuer. *J. Amer. Chem. Soc.* **96**, 2246 (1974).

181. S. Hirase, S. Nakai, T. Akatsu, A. Kobayashi, M. Oohara, K-I. Matsunaga, M. Fujii, S. Kodaira, T. Fujii, T. Furusho, Y. Ohmura, T. Wada, C. Yoshikumi, S. Ueno, and S. Ohtsuka. *Yakugaku Zasshi* **96**, 413 (1976).
182. J. J. Hoffmann, S. J. Torrance, R. M. Wiedhopf, and J. R. Cole. *J. Pharm. Sci.* **66**, 883 (1977).
183. J. J. Hoffmann, R. M. Wiedhopf, and J. R. Cole. *J. Pharm. Sci.* **66**, 586 (1977).
184. W. Hofheinz and W. O. Operhänsli. *Helv. Chim. Acta* **60**, 660 (1977).
185. W. Hofheinz and P. Schönholzer. *Helv. Chim. Acta* **60**, 1367 (1977).
186. K. Horáková, B. Kernáčová, P. Nemec, and J. Fuska. *J. Antibiot. Tokyo* **29** 1109 (1976).
187. D. H. S. Horn, S. Fabbri, F. Hampshire, and M. E. Lowe. *Biochem. J.* **109**, 399 (1968).
188. D. H. S. Horn, E. J. Middleton, J. A. Wunderlich, and F. Hampshire. *J.C.S. Chem. Commun.* 339 (1966).
189. M. B. Hossain, A. F. Nicholas, D. Van Der Helm. *J.C.S. Chem. Commun.* 385 (1968).
190. M. B. Hossain, D. Van Der Helm. *Rec. Trav. Chim. Pays-Bas* **88**, 1413 (1969).
191. L. H. Hurley. *J. Antibiot. Tokyo* **30**, 349 (1977).
192. D. R. Idler and U. H. M. Fagerlund. *J. Amer. Chem. Soc.* **77**, 4142 (1955).
193. D. R. Idler and P. Wiseman. *Comp. Biochem. Physiol.* **26**, 1113 (1968).
194. D. R. Idler, P. M. Wiseman, and L. M. Safe. *Steroids* **16**, 451 (1970).
195. A. Iengo, L. Mayol, and C. Santacroce. *Experientia* **33**, 11 (1977).
196. S. Ikegami, Y. Kamiya, and S. Tamura. *Tetrahedron Lett.* 731 (1973).
197. S. Ikegami, Y. Kamiya, and S. Tamura. *Tetrahedron Lett.* 3725 (1972).
198. S. Ikegami, Y. Kamiya, and S. Tamura. *Tetrahedron Lett.* 1601 (1972).
199. C. Ireland and D. J. Faulkner. *J. Org. Chem.* **42**, 3157 (1977).
200. M. Isemura and T. Ikenaka. *Experientia* **33**, 871 (1977).
201. K. Isono. *J. Antibiot. Tokyo Ser. A* **14**, 160 (1961).
202. H. Ito and M. Sugiura. *Chem. Pharm. Bull. Tokyo* **24**, 1114 (1976).
203. H. Ito, M. Sugiura, and T. Miyazaki. *Chem. Pharm. Bull. Tokyo* **24**, 2575 (1976).
204. S. Ito and Y. Hirata. *Tetrahedron Lett.* 2429 (1977).
205. R. W. Jeanloz, A. K. Bhattacharyya, and G. P. Roberts. *Hoppe-Seylers Z. Physiol. Chem.* **350**, 663 (1969).
206. J. Jizba, V. Herout, and F. Šorm. *Tetrahedron Lett.* 1689 (1967).
207. S. Jolad, J. J. Hoffmann, R. M. Wiedhopf, J. R. Cole, R. B. Bates, and G. R. Kriek. *Tetrahedron Lett.* 4119 (1976).
208. S. D. Jolad, R. M. Wiedhopf, and J. R. Cole. *J. Pharm. Sci.* **66**, 892 (1977).
209. S. D. Jolad, R. M. Wiedhopf, and J. R. Cole. *J. Pharm. Sci.* **66**, 889 (1977).
210. M. Kaisin, Y. M. Sheikh, L. J. Durham, C. Djerassi, B. Tursch, D. Daloze, J. C. Braekman, D. Losman, and R. Karlsson. *Tetrahedron Lett.* 2239 (1974).
211. Y. Kamiya, S. Ikegami, and S. Tamura. *Tetrahedron Lett.* 655 (1974).
212. N. Kaneda, T. Sasaki, and K. Hayashi. *Protein Structure* **491**, 53 (1977).
213. J. Karnetová, J. Mateju, P. Sedmera, J. Vokoun, and Z. Vanek. *J. Antibiot. Tokyo* **29**, 1199 (1976).
214. Y. Kashman and A. Groweiss. *Tetrahedron Lett.* 1159 (1977).
215. Y. Kashman, E. Zadock, and I. Néeman. *Tetrahedron* **30**, 3615 (1974).
216. T. Katayama, K. Shintani, and C. O. Chichester. *Comp. Biochem. Physiol.* **44B**, 253 (1973).
217. T. Katayama, H. Yokoyama, and C. O. Chichester. *Int. J. Biochem.* **1**, 438 (1970).
218. T. Katayama, H. Yokoyama, and C. O. Chichester. *Bull. Jap. Soc. Sci. Fish.* **36**, 702 (1970).
219. Y. Kato and P. J. Scheuer. *Pure Appl. Chem.* **41**, 1 (1975).
220. Y. Kato and P. J. Scheuer. *J. Amer. Chem. Soc.* **96**, 2245 (1974).

221. R. L. Katzman, M. H. Halford, V. N. Reinhold, and R. W. Jeanloz. *Biochemistry* **11**, 1161 (1972).
221a. P. N. Kaul, S. K. Kulkarni, A. J. Weinheimer, F. J. Schmitz, and T. K. B. Karns. *J. Nat. Prod.* **40**, 253 (1977).
222. R. Kazlauskas, P. T. Murphy, R. J. Quinn, and R. J. Wells. *Tetrahedron Lett.* 61 (1977).
223. R. Kazlauskas, P. T. Murphy, R. J. Quinn, and R. J. Wells. *Tetrahedron Lett.* 2635 (1976).
224. R. Kazlauskas, P. T. Murphy, R. J. Quinn, and R. J. Wells. *Tetrahedron Lett.* 2631 (1976).
225. A. Kelecom, D. Daloze, and B. Tursch. *Tetrahedron* **32**, 2353 (1976).
226. A. Kelecom, D. Daloze, and B. Tursch. *Tetrahedron* **32**, 2313 (1976).
227. W. R. Kem, B. C. Abbott, and R. M. Coates. *Toxicon* **9**, 15 (1971).
228. O. Kennard, D. G. Watson, L. R. di Sanseverino, B. Tursch, R. Bosmans, and C. Djerassi. *Tetrahedron Lett.* 2879 (1968).
229. R. A. Kent, I. R. Smith, and M. D. Sutherland. *Aust. J. Chem.* **23**, 2325 (1970).
230. C. A. Kind and R. A. Meigs. *J. Org. Chem.* **20**, 1116 (1955).
231. D. G. I. Kingston, F. Ionescu, and B. T. Li. *Lloydia* **40**, 215 (1977).
232. D. G. I. Kingston, B. T. Li, and F. Ionescu. *J. Pharm. Sci.* **66**, 1135 (1977).
233. V. V. Kiselev. *Chem. Nat. Comp. USSR* **13**, 1 (1977).
234. Y. Kishi, H. Tanino, and T. Goto. *Tetrahedron Lett.* 2747 (1972).
235. I. Kitagawa and M. Kobayashi. *Tetrahedron Lett.* 859 (1977).
236. I. Kitagawa, M. Kobayashi, T. Sugawara, and I. Yosioka. *Tetrahedron Lett.* 967 (1975).
237. I. Kitagawa, T. Sugawara, and I. Yosioka. *Tetrahedron Lett.* 4111 (1974).
238. I. Kitagawa, T. Sugawara, I. Yosioka, and K. Kuriyama. *Tetrahedron Lett.* 963 (1975).
239. T. Kitahara, H. Naganawa, T. Okazaki, Y. Okami, and H. Umezawa. *J. Antibiot. Tokyo* **28**, 280 (1975).
240. J. S. Kittredge and R. R. Hughes. *Biochemistry* **3**, 991 (1964).
241. J. S. Kittredge, A. F. Isbell, and R. R. Hughes. *Biochemistry* **6**, 289 (1967).
242. J. S. Kittredge, E. Roberts, and D. G. Simonsen. *Biochemistry* **1**, 624 (1962).
243. E. S. Kline and H. Weissbach. *Life Sci.* **4**, 63 (1965).
244. M. Kobayashi and H. Mitsuhashi. *Steroids* **24**, 399 (1974).
245. M. Kobayashi and H. Mitsuhashi. *Tetrahedron* **30**, 2147 (1974).
246. M. Kobayashi, M. Nishizawa, K. Todo, and H. Mitsuhashi. *Chem. Pharm. Bull. Tokyo* **21**, 323 (1973).
247. M. Kobayashi, R. Tsuru, K. Todo, and H. Mitsuhashi. *Tetrahedron* **29**, 1193 (1973).
248. M. Kobayashi, R. Tsuru, K. Todo, and H. Mitsuhashi. *Tetrahedron Lett.* 2935 (1972).
249. K. Komiyama, K. Sugimoto, H. Takeshima, and I. Umezawa. *J. Antibiot. Tokyo* **30**, 202 (1977).
250. Y. Komoda, S. Kaneko, M. Yamamoto, M. Ishikawa, A. Itai, and Y. Iitaka. *Chem. Pharm. Bull. Tokyo* **23**, 2464 (1975).
251. T. Kosuge, H. Zenda, A. Ochiai, N. Masaki, M. Noguchi, S. Kimura, and H. Narita. *Tetrahedron Lett.* 2545 (1972).
252. G. E. Krejcarek, R. H. White, L. P. Hager, W. O. McClure, R. D. Johnson, K. L. Rinehart, Jr., J. A. McMillan, I. C. Paul, P. D. Shaw, and R. C. Brusca. *Tetrahedron Lett.* 507 (1975).
253. D. Kritchevsky, S. A. Tepper, N. W. DiTullo, and W. L. Holmes. *J. Food Sci.* **32**, 64 (1967).
254. R. Kuhn and K. Wallenfels. *Chem. Ber.* **72**, 1407 (1939).
255. S. M. Kupchan. *Cancer Treatment Reports* **60**, 1115 (1976).

256. S. M. Kupchan, B. B. Jarvis, R. G. Dailey, Jr., W. Bright, R. F. Bryan, and Y. Shizuri. *J. Amer. Chem. Soc.* **98**, 7092 (1976).
257. S. M. Kupchan and A. Karim. *Lloydia* **39**, 223 (1976).
258. S. M. Kupchan and H. L. Kopperman. *Experientia* **31**, 625 (1975).
259. S. M. Kupchan, E. J. LaVoie, A. R. Branfman, B. Y. Fei, W. M. Bright, and R. F. Bryan. *J. Amer. Chem. Soc.* **99**, 3199 (1977).
260. S. M. Kupchan, Y. Shizuri, T. Murae, J. G. Sweeny, H. R. Haynes, M-S. Shen, J. C. Barrick, R. F. Bryan, D. van Der Helm, and K. K. Wu. *J. Amer. Chem. Soc.* **98**, 5719 (1976).
261. S. M. Kupchan, Y. Shizuri, W. C. Sumner, Jr., H. R. Haynes, A. P. Leighton, and B. R. Sickles. *J. Org. Chem.* **41**, 3850 (1976).
262. S. M. Kupchan and D. R. Streelman. *J. Org. Chem.* **41**, 3481 (1976).
263. H. Kuroda, S. Nakazawa, K. Katagiri, O. Shiratori, M. Kozuka, K. Fujitani, and M. Tomita. *Chem. Pharm. Bull. Tokyo* **24**, 2413 (1976).
264. J. P. Kutney. *Lloydia* **40**, 107 (1977).
265. J. P. Kutney, J. Balsevich, and G. H. Bokelman. *Heterocycles* **4**, 1377 (1976).
266. J. P. Kutney, J. Balsevich, G. H. Bokelman, T. Hibino, I. Itoh, and A. H. Ratcliffe. *Heterocycles* **4**, 997 (1976).
267. J. P. Kutney, G. H. Bokelman, M. Ichikawa, E. Jahngen, A. V. Joshua, P-H. Liao, and B. R. Worth. *Heterocycles* **4**, 1267 (1976).
268. J. P. Kutney, T. Hibino, E. Jahngen, T. Okutani, A. H. Ratcliffe, A. M. Treasurywala, and S. Wunderly. *Helv. Chim. Acta* **59**, 2858 (1976).
269. J. P. Kutney, E. Jahngen, and T. Okutani. *Heterocycles* **5**, 59 (1976).
270. J. P. Kutney and B. R. Worth. *Heterocycles* **4**, 1777 (1976).
271. W. L. Lasswell, Jr. and C. D. Hufford. *J. Org. Chem.* **42**, 1295 (1977).
272. K-H. Lee, I. H. Hall, E-C. Mar, C. O. Starnes, S. A. El Gebaly, T. G. Waddell, R. I. Hadgraft, C. G. Ruffner, and I. Weidner. *J. Sci.* **196**, 533 (1977).
273. K-H. Lee, M. Haruna, H-C. Huang, B-S. Wu, and I. H. Hall, *J. Pharm. Sci.* **66** 1194 (1977).
274. K-H. Lee, Y. Imakura, and D. Sims. *J. Pharm. Sci.* **65**, 1410 (1976).
275. K-H. Lee, Y. Imakura, D. Sims, A. T. McPhail, and K. D. Onan. *Phytochemistry* **16**, 393 (1977).
276. W. W. Lee, A. Benitez, L. Goodman, and B. R. Baker. *J. Amer. Chem. Soc.* **82**, 2648 (1960).
277. T. L. Lentz. *J. Exp. Zool.* **162**, 171 (1966).
278. P. W. LeQuesne, M. P. Pastore, and R. F. Raffauf. *Lloydia* **39**, 391 (1976).
279. L. H. Li, S. L. Kuentzel, K. D. Shugars, and B. K. Bhuyan. *J. Antibiot. Tokyo* **30**, 506 (1977).
280. N. C. Ling, R. L. Hale, and C. Djerassi. *J. Amer. Chem. Soc.* **92**, 5281 (1970).
281. A. W. Lis, R. K. McLaughlin, D. I. McLaughlin, G. D. Daves, Jr., and W. R. Anderson, Jr. *J. Amer. Chem. Soc.* **95**, 5789 (1973).
282. E. M. Low. *J. Marine Res.* **10**, 239 (1951).
283. S. Makisumi. *J. Biochem. Tokyo* **49**, 284 (1961).
284. F. B. Mallory, J. T. Gordon, and R. L. Conner. *J. Amer. Chem. Soc.* **85**, 1362 (1963).
285. P. S. Manchand and J. F. Blount. *Tetrahedron Lett.* 2489 (1976).
286. D. G. Martin, C. G. Chidester, S. A. Mizsak, D. J. Duchamp, L. Baczynskyj, W. C. Krueger, R. J. Wnuk, and P. A. Meulman. *J. Antibiot. Tokyo* **28**, 91 (1975).
287. A. P. Mathias, D. M. Ross, and M. Schachter. *J. Physiol. London* **142**, 56p (1958).
288. J. W. Mathieson and R. H. Thomson. *J. Chem. Soc. (C)*, 153 (1971).
289. H. Matsuda, Y. Tomiie, S. Yamamura, and Y. Hirata. *J.C.S. Chem. Commun.* 898 (1967).
290. T. Matsuno and T. Ito. *Experientia* **27**, 509 (1971).

291. F. J. McDonald, D. C. Campbell, D. J. Vanderah, F. J. Schmitz, D. M. Washecheck, J. E. Burks, and D. Van Der Helm. *J. Org. Chem.* **40**, 665 (1975).
292. D. H. Miles, J. Bhattacharyya, N. V. Mody, J. L. Atwood, S. Black, and P. A. Hedin. *J. Amer. Chem. Soc.* **99**, 618 (1977).
293. L. Minale. *Pure Appl. Chem.* **48**, 7 (1976).
294. L. Minale, G. Cimino, S. De Stefano, and G. Sodano. *Forschritte Chem. Org. Naturst.* **33**, 1 (1976).
295. L. Minale and R. Riccio. *Tetrahedron Lett.* 2711 (1976).
296. L. Minale, R. Riccio, and G. Sodano. *Tetrahedron* **30**, 1341 (1974).
297. L. Minale, R. Riccio, and G. Sodano. *Tetrahedron Lett.* 3401 (1974).
298. L. Minale and G. Sodano. *J.C.S. Perkin Trans I* 2380 (1974).
299. L. Minale and G. Sodano. *J.C.S. Perkin Trans I* 1888 (1974).
300. L. Minale, G. Sodano, W. R. Chan, and A. M. Chen. *J.C.S. Chem. Commun.* 674 (1972).
301. M. G. Missakian, B. J. Burreson, and P. J. Scheuer. *Tetrahedron* **31**, 2513 (1975).
302. J. M. Moldowan, W. L. Tan, and C. Djerassi. *Steroids* **26**, 107 (1975).
303. J. M. Moldowan, B. M. Tursch, and C. Djerassi. *Steroids* **24**, 387 (1974).
304. R. Montgomery, F. Yamauchi, and W. T. Bradner. *Lloydia* **40**, 269 (1977).
305. K. Moody, R. H. Thomson, E. Fattorusso, L. Minale, and G. Sodano. *J.C.S. Perkin Trans.* **I** 18 (1972).
306. H. W. Moore. *Science* **197**, 527 (1977).
307. R. E. Moore, H. Singh, and P. J. Scheuer. *Tetrahedron Lett.* 4581 (1968).
308. R. E. Moore, H. Singh, and P. J. Scheuer. *J. Org. Chem.* **31**, 3645 (1966).
309. I. Morimoto, M. I. N. Shaikh, R. H. Thomson, and D. G. Williamson. *J.C.S. Chem. Commun.* 550 (1970).
310. T. Mukai. *Bull. Chem. Soc. Jap.* **33**, 1234 (1960).
311. T. Mukai. *Bull. Chem. Soc. Jap.* **33**, 453 (1960).
312. I. Ne'eman, L. Fishelson, and Y. Kashman. *Toxicon* **12**, 593 (1974).
313. D. E. Nettleton, Jr., W. T. Bradner, J. A. Bush, A. B. Coon, J. E. Moseley, R. W. Myllymaki, F. A. O'Herron, R. H. Schreiber, and A. L. Vulcano. *J. Antibiot. Tokyo* **30**, 525 (1977).
314. T. Noguchi, S. Konosu, and Y. Hashimoto. *Toxicon* **7**, 325 (1969).
315. T. R. Norton, S. Shibata, M. Kashiwagi, and J. Bentley. *J. Pharm. Sci.* **65**, 1368 (1976).
316. M. Ogura, G. A. Cordell, and N. R. Farnsworth. *Lloydia* **40**, 157 (1977).
317. M. Ogura, G. A. Cordell, and N. R. Farnsworth. *Lloydia* **39**, 255 (1976).
318. Y. Ogura and Y. Mori. *Eur. J. Pharmacol.* **3**, 58 (1968).
319. T. Okaichi and Y. Hashimoto. *Agr. Biol. Chem. Tokyo* **26**, 224 (1962).
320. Y. Okami, T. Okazaki, T. Kitahara, and H. Umezawa. *J. Antibiot. Tokyo* **29** 1019 (1976).
321. R. Pal, D. K. Kulshreshtha, and R. P. Rastogi. *J. Pharm. Sci.* **65**, 918 (1976).
322. L. A. Pavelka, Y. H. Kim, and H. S. Mosher. *Toxicon* **15**, 135 (1977).
323. Th. Payne and S. S. Kuwahara. *Experientia* **28**, 1022 (1972).
324. G. R. Pettit. *Biosynthetic Products for Cancer Chemotherapy*, *Vol. 1*, Plenum Publishing Corp., New York, N.Y., 1977, p. 146.
325. G. R. Pettit. *Biosynthetic Products for Cancer Chemotherapy*, *Vol. 1*, Plenum Publishing Corp., New York, N.Y., 1977, pp. 50, 165, 177.
326. G. R. Pettit. *Synthetic Peptides, Vol.1*, Van Nostrand Reinhold Co., New York, N.Y., 1970, p. 380.
327. G. R. Pettit, R. M. Blazer, and D. A. Reierson. *Lloydia* **40**, 247 (1977).
328. G. R. Pettit, J. C. Budzinski, G. M. Cragg, P. Brown, and L. D. Johnston. *J. Med. Chem.* **17**, 1013 (1974).
329. G. R. Pettit and G. M. Cragg. *Biosynthetic Products for Cancer Chemotherapy*, *Vol. 2*, Plenum Publishing Corp., New York, N.Y., 1978.

330. G. R. Pettit and G. M. Cragg. *Experientia* **29**, 781 (1973).
331. G. R. Pettit and D. L. Doubek, unpublished experiments.
332. G. R. Pettit and C. L. Herald, unpublished experiments.
333. G. R. Pettit, C. L. Herald, J. J. Einck, L. D. Vanell, P. Brown, and D. Gust. *J. Org. Chem.*, in press.
334. G. R. Pettit, C. L. Herald, and D. L. Herald. *J. Pharm. Sci.* **65**, 1558 (1976).
335. G. R. Pettit, C. L. Herald, and R. H. Ode, unpublished experiments.
336. G. R. Pettit, C. L. Herald, R. H. Ode, and L. D. Vanell, unpublished experiments.
337. G. R. Pettit, C. L. Herald, L. D. Vanell, R. H. Ode, M. S. Allen, D. L. Herald, and J. F. Day, unpublished experiments.
338. G. R. Pettit and R. H. Ode. *J. Pharm. Sci.* **66**, 757 (1977).
339. G. R. Pettit, R. H. Ode, and T. B. Harvey, III. *Lloydia* **36**, 204 (1973).
340. G. R. Pettit, R. B. Von Dreele, G. Bolliger, P. M. Traxler, and P. Brown. *Experientia* **29**, 521 (1973).
341. S. Popov, R. M. K. Carlson, A. Wegmann, and C. Djerassi. *Steroids* **28**, 699 (1976).
342. S. Popov, R. M. K. Carlson, A-M. Wegmann, and C. Djerassi. *Tetrahedron Lett.* 3491 (1976).
343. V. H. Powell and M. D. Sutherland. *Aust. J. Chem.* **20**, 541 (1967).
344. V. H. Powell, M. D. Sutherland, and J. W. Wells. *Aust. J. Chem.* **20**, 535 (1967).
345. G. Prota, M. D'Agostino, and G. Misuraca. *J.C.S. Perkin Trans I* 1614 (1972).
346. L. D. Quin. *Science* **144**, 1133 (1964).
347. W. D. Raverty, R. H. Thomson, and T. J. King. *J.C.S. Perkin Trans I* 1204 (1977).
348. J. Roche, Y. Robin, N-V. Thoai, and L. A. Pradel. *Comp. Biochem. Physiol.* **1**, 44 (1960).
349. P. Roller, C. Djerassi, R. Cloetens, and B. Tursch. *J. Amer. Chem. Soc.* **91**, 4918 (1969).
350. I. Rothberg, B. M. Tursch, and C. Djerassi. *J. Org. Chem.* **38**, 209 (1973).
351. W. Rüdiger, W. Klose, B. Tursch, N. Houvenaghel-Crevecoeur, and H. Budzikiewicz. *Justus Liebigs Ann. Chem.* **713**, 209 (1968).
352. G. D. Ruggieri. *Science* **194**, 491 (1976).
353. A. A. Saleh, G. A. Cordell, and N. R. Farnsworth. *Lloydia* **39**, 456 (1976).
354. A. W. Sangster, S. E. Thomas, and N. L. Tingling. *Tetrahedron* **31**, 1135 (1975).
355. M. G. Santoro, G. W. Philpott, and B. M. Jaffe. *Nature* **263**, 777 (1976).
356. I. V. E. Savage and M. E. H. Howden. *Toxicon* **15**, 463 (1977).
357. F. M. Schabel, Jr. *Chemotherapy* **13**, 321 (1968).
358. E. J. Schantz, V. E. Ghazarossian, H. K. Schnoes, F. M. Strong, J. P. Springer, J. O. Pezzanite, and J. Clardy. *J. Amer. Chem. Soc.* **97**, 1238 (1975).
359. E. J. Schantz, J. M. Lynch, G. Vayvada, K. Matsumoto, and H. Rapoport. *Biochemistry* **5**, 1191 (1966).
360. P. J. Scheuer. *Account Chem. Res.* **10**, 33 (1977).
361. P. J. Scheuer. *Chemistry of Marine Natural Products*, Academic Press, New York, 1973.
362. H. Schildknecht, H. Neumaier, and B. Tauscher. *Justus Liebigs Ann. Chem.* **756**, 155 (1972).
363. F. J. Schmitz, K. W. Kraus, L. S. Ciereszko, D. H. Sifford, and A. J. Weinheimer. *Tetrahedron Lett.* 97 (1966).
364. F. J. Schmitz and E. D. Lorance. *J. Org. Chem.* **36**, 719 (1971).
365. F. J. Schmitz, E. D. Lorance, and L. S. Ciereszko. *J. Org. Chem.* **34**, 1989 (1969).
366. F. J. Schmitz and F. J. McDonald. *Tetrahedron Lett.* 2541 (1974).
367. F. J. Schmitz and T. Pattabhiraman. *J. Amer. Chem. Soc.* **92**, 6073 (1970).

368. F. J. Schmitz, D. J. Vanderah, and L. S. Ciereszko. *J.C.S. Chem. Commun.* 407 (1974).
369. W. P. Schneider, R. D. Hamilton, and L. E. Rhuland. *J. Amer. Chem. Soc.* **94**, 2122 (1972).
370. W. P. Schneider, R. A. Morge, and B. E. Henson. *J. Amer. Chem. Soc.* **99**, 6062 (1977).
371. W. Schuett and H. Rapoport. *J. Amer. Chem. Soc.* **84**, 2266 (1962).
372. S. Sekita, K. Yoshihira, S. Natori, and H. Kuwano. *Tetrahedron Lett.* 1351 (1976)
373. G. M. Sharma and P. R. Burkholder. *J.C.S. Chem. Commun.* 151 (1971).
374. G. M. Sharma and P. R. Burkholder. *J. Antibiot. Tokyo Ser. A* **20**, 200 (1967).
375. G. M. Sharma and P. R. Burkholder. *Tetrahedron Lett.* 4147 (1967).
376. G. M. Sharma and B. Vig. *Tetrahedron Lett.* 1715 (1972).
377. G. M. Sharma, B. Vig, and P. R. Burkholder. *J. Org. Chem.* **35**, 2823 (1970).
378. Y. M. Sheikh and C. Djerassi. *Tetrahedron Lett.* 3111 (1977).
379. Y. M. Sheikh and C. Djerassi. *J.C.S. Chem. Commun.* 1057 (1976).
380. Y. M. Sheikh and C. Djerassi. *Experientia* **31**, 265 (1975).
381. Y. M. Sheikh and C. Djerassi. *Tetrahedron* **30**, 4095 (1974).
382. Y. M. Sheikh and C. Djerassi. *Tetrahedron Lett.* 2927 (1973).
383. Y. M. Sheikh, C. Djerassi, J. C. Braekman, D. Daloze, M. Kaisin, B. Tursch, and R. Karlsson. *Tetrahedron* **33**, 2115 (1977).
384. Y. M. Sheikh, C. Djerassi, and B. M. Tursch. *J.C.S. Chem. Commun.* 600 (1971).
385. Y. M. Sheikh, C. Djerassi, and B. M. Tursch. *J.C.S. Chem. Commun.* 217 (1971).
386. Y. M. Sheikh, B. Tursch, and C. Djerassi. *Tetrahedron Lett.* 3721 (1972).
387. O. Shimomura, T. Goto, and Y. Hirata. *Bull. Chem. Soc. Jap.* **30**, 929 (1957).
388. M. M. Sigel, W. Lichter, L. L. Wellham, and D. M. Lopez. "Cytotoxic and Antiproliferative Substances in Invertebrates and Poikilothermic Vertebrates," in *Invertebrate Tissue Culture. Applications in Medicine, Biology, and Agriculture*, Academic Press, Inc., 1976, p. 309.
389. H. Singh, R. E. Moore, and P. J. Scheuer. *Experientia* **23**, 624 (1967).
390. I. Singh, R. T. Ogata, R. E. Moore, C. W. J. Chang, and P. J. Scheuer. *Tetrahedron* **24**, 6053 (1968).
391. J. F. Siuda. *Lloydia* **37**, 501 (1974).
392. H. L. Sleeper and W. Fenical. *J. Amer. Chem. Soc.* **99**, 2367 (1977).
393. C. R. Smith, Jr., R. G. Powell, and K. L. Mikolajczak. *Cancer Treatment Reports* **60**, 1157 (1976).
394. D. S. H. Smith, A. B. Turner, and A. M. Mackie. *J.C.S. Perkin Trans I* 1745 (1973).
395. I. R. Smith and M. D. Sutherland. *Aust. J. Chem.* **24**, 1487 (1971).
396. J. Smith and R. H. Thomson. *Tetrahedron Lett.* 10 (1960).
397. R. W. Spjut and R. E. Perdue, Jr. *Cancer Treatment Reports* **60**, 979 (1976).
398. J. P. Springer, J. Clardy, J. M. Wells, R. J. Cole, J. W. Kirksey, R. D. Macfarlane, and D. F. Torgerson. *Tetrahedron Lett.* 1355 (1976).
399. J. H. Songdahl and B. I. Shapiro. *Toxicon* **12**, 109 (1974).
400. E. Steiner, C. Djerassi, E. Fattorusso, S. Magno, L. Mayol, C. Santacroce, and D. Sica. *Helv. Chim. Acta* **60**, 475 (1977).
401. H. H. Strain, W. A. Svec, K. Aitzetmüller, M. C. Grandolfo, J. J. Katz, H. Kjøsen, S. Norgard, S. Liaaen-Jensen, F. T. Haxo, P. Wegfahrt, and H. Rapoport. *J. Amer. Chem. Soc.* **93**, 1823 (1971).
402. R. J. Suhadolnik. "Spongosine and Arabinosyl Nucleosides," in *Nucleoside Antibiotics*, Wiley-Interscience, N.Y., 1970, p. 123.
403. Y. Sumiki, K. Isono, J. Nagatsu, and T. Takauchi. *J. Antibiot. Tokyo Ser A.* **13**, 416 (1960).
404. M. D. Sutherland and J. W. Wells. *Aust. J. Chem.* **20**, 515 (1967).

405. S. Tafur, J. D. Nelson, D. C. DeLong, and G. H. Svoboda. *Lloydia* **39**, 261 (1976).
406. B. Tammami, S. J. Torrance, and J. R. Cole. *Phytochemistry* **16**, 1100 (1977).
407. T. Tamura, T. Wainai, B. Truscott, and D. R. Idler. *Can. J. Biochem. Physiol.* **42**, 1331 (1964).
408. W. L. Tan, C. Djerassi, J. Fayos, and J. Clardy. *J. Org. Chem.* **40**, 466 (1975).
409. S. J. Torrance, R. M. Wiedhopf, J. R. Cole, S. K. Arora, R. B. Bates, W. A. Beavers, and R. S. Cutler. *J. Org. Chem.* **41**, 1855 (1976).
410. E. R. Trumbull, E. Bianchi, D. J. Eckert, R. M. Wiedhopf, and J. R. Cole. *J. Pharm. Sci.* **65**, 1407 (1976).
411. B. Tursch, J. C. Braekman, and D. Daloze. *Bull. Soc. Chim. Belg.* **84**, 767 (1975).
412. B. Tursch, J. C. Braekman, D. Daloze, P. Fritz, A. Kelecom, R. Karlsson, and D. Losman. *Tetrahedron Lett.* 747 (1974).
413. B. Tursch, J. C. Braekman, D. Daloze, M. Herin, and R. Karlsson. *Tetrahedron Lett.* 3769 (1974).
414. B. Tursch, J. C. Braekman, D. Daloze, M. Herin, R. Karlsson, and D. Losman. *Tetrahedron* **31**, 129 (1975).
415. B. Tursch, R. Cloetens, and C. Djerassi. *Tetrahedron Lett.* 467 (1970).
416. B. Tursch, I. S. DeSouza Guimarães, B. Gilbert, R. T. Aplin, A. M. Duffield, and C. Djerassi. *Tetrahedron* **23**, 761 (1967).
417. Y. Ueno, et. al. *Proc. Jap. Acad.* **33**, 53 (1957).
418. H. Umezawa. *Lloydia* **40**, 67 (1977).
419. I. Umezawa, K. Komiyama, H. Takeshima, J. Awaya, and S. Ōmura. *J. Antibiot. Tokyo* **29**, 1249 (1976).
420. D. J. Vanderah and C. Djerassi. *Tetrahedron Lett.* 683 (1977).
421. D. J. Vanderah and F. J. Schmitz. *J. Org. Chem.* **41**, 3480 (1976).
422. D. J. Vanderah and F. J. Schmitz. *Lloydia* **38**, 271 (1975).
423. D. J. Vanderah, P. A. Steudler, L. S. Ciereszko, F. J. Schmitz, J. D. Ekstrand, and D. Van Der Helm. *J. Amer. Chem. Soc.* **99**, 5780 (1977).
424. G. E. Van Lear, G. O. Morton, and W. Fulmor. *Tetrahedron Lett.* 299 (1973).
425. M. E. Wall, M. C. Wani, and H. Taylor. *Cancer Treatment Reports* **60**, 1011 (1976).
426. M. C. Wani, H. L. Taylor, and M. E. Wall. *J.C.S. Chem. Commun.* 295 (1977).
427. A. J. Weinheimer, T. K. B. Karns, D. H. Sifford, and L. S. Ciereszko. *Amer. Chem. Soc. Abstr.* P171 (1968).
428. A. J. Weinheimer, J. A. Matson, M. B. Hossain, and D. Van Der Helm. *Tetrahedron Lett.* 2923 (1977).
429. A. J. Weinheimer, J. A. Matson, D. Van Der Helm, and M. Poling. *Tetrahedron Lett.* 1295 (1977).
430. A. J. Weinheimer, E. K. Metzner, and M. L. Mole, Jr. *Tetrahedron* **29**, 3135 (1973).
431. A. J. Weinheimer, R. E. Middlebrook, J. O. Bledsoe, Jr., W. E. Marsico, and T. K. B. Karns. *J.C.S. Chem. Commun.* 384 (1968).
432. A. J. Weinheimer and R. L. Spraggins. *Tetrahedron Lett.* 5185 (1969).
433. A. J. Weinheimer and P. H. Washecheck. *Tetrahedron Lett.* 3315 (1969).
434. A. J. Weinheimer, P. H. Washecheck, D. Van Der Helm, and M. B. Hossain. *J.C.S. Chem. Commun.* 1070 (1968).
435. A. J. Weinheimer, W. W. Youngblood, P. H. Washecheck, T. K. B. Karns, and L. S. Ciereszko. *Tetrahedron Lett.* 497 (1970).
436. B. S. Welinder. *Biochim. Biophys. Acta.* **279**, 491 (1972).
437. R. J. Wells. *Tetrahedron Lett.* 2637 (1976).
438. H. L. Wheeler and L. B. Mendel. *J. Biol. Chem.* **7**, 1 (1909).
439. R. J. Whitley, S-J. Soong, R. Bolin, G. J. Galasso, L. T. Ch'ien, and C. A. Alford. *N. Engl. J. Med.* **297**, 289 (1977).

440. P. F. Wiley. *J. Antibiot. Tokyo* **29**, 587 (1976).
441. P. F. Wiley, R. B. Kelly, E. L. Caron, V. H. Wiley, J. H. Johnson, F. A. MacKellar, and S. A. Mizsak. *J. Amer. Chem. Soc.* **99**, 542 (1977).
442. M. Williams and J. M. Cassady. *J. Pharm. Sci.* **65**, 912 (1976).
443. J. L. Wong, R. Oesterlin, and H. Rapoport. *J. Amer. Chem. Soc.* **93**, 7344 (1971).
444. J. G. Wood and T. L. Lentz. *Nature* **201**, 88 (1964).
445. S. J. Wratten, D. J. Faulkner, K. Hirotsu, and J. Clardy. *J. Amer. Chem. Soc.* **99**, 2824 (1977).
446. S. J. Wratten, W. Fenical, D. J. Faulkner, and J. C. Wekell. *Tetrahedron Lett.* 1559 (1977).
447. M. Yamagushi. *Bull. Chem. Soc. Jap.* **32**, 1171 (1959).
448. M. Yamaguchi. *Bull. Chem. Soc. Jap.* **31**, 739 (1958).
449. M. Yamaguchi. *Bull. Chem. Soc. Jap.* **31**, 51 (1958).
450. M. Yamaguchi. *Bull. Chem. Soc. Jap.* **30**, 979 (1957).
451. M. Yamaguchi. *Bull. Chem. Soc. Jap.* **30**, 111 (1957).
452. S. Yamamura and Y. Hirata. *Bull. Chem. Soc. Jap.* **44**, 2560 (1971).
453. S. Yamamura and Y. Hirata. *Tetrahedron* **19**, 1485 (1963).
454. S. Yamamura and Y. Terada. *Tetrahedron Lett.* 2171 (1977).
455. Y. Yasmmoto, T. Watanabe, and Y. Hashimoto. *Bull. Jap. Soc. Sci. Fish.* **30** 357 (1964).
456. S. Yasuda. *Comp. Biochem. Physiol.* **44B**, 41 (1973).